THE COMPLETE BOOK OF CYCLOCROSS
Skill Training and Racing

Scott Mares

SIBEX SPORTS
Colorado Springs, Colorado

For more information:
www.sibexsports.com
www.cx-book.com

ISBN: 0-6152248-5-7

Printed in the United States of America.

5 4 3 2

Table of Contents

About the Author

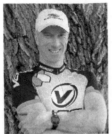 Scott Mares was born in Oklahoma City, Oklahoma and started racing his bicycle when he was in high school. Scott was an active racer in the community throughout his junior years. Scott attended New Mexico Military Institute and graduated with a Liberal Arts degree and went on to the University of Oklahoma to earn a BS in Health and Sports Sciences with a minor in Microbiology. While attending the University of Oklahoma, Scott was a Pulmonary Function Tech and working in the Pulmonary Function Blood Gas Lab at University Hospital in Oklahoma City. After graduation, he became a Certified Strength and Conditioning Specialist. He also was a cyclocross athlete at the United States Olympic Training Center, Colorado Springs, in 1994, and in 1996 he completed an internship for the USAC during the Atlanta Games Super Camp. After graduation, Scott moved became part of the cycling community in Colorado Springs.

After racing cross in Colorado, he put together local clinics for his cycling buddies in cyclocross and the word quickly got out about his skill drills. Scott then received a call from his friend Jim Copeland to come and help at the first ACA Jr. Cyclocross camp in Deckers, Colorado. Jim asked Scott to come and coach, but at the time, he focused only on teaching skill. Jim Copeland told him, "That's perfect!" Scott showed up to camp that morning and Jim informed Scott that he was in charge. At the time of publication of this book, Scott was the head coach at cyclocross camp for nine straight years. The cyclocross camps were free to kids and started out with 50 juniors. By 2007, there were over 140 kids, making it the largest junior cyclocross camp in the world.

In 1999, Scott was having coffee with his coach and wanted a Titanium cyclocross bike. His coach told him that he had an athlete in the Moscow Embassy that knew where the factory was. This meeting eventually spawned the beginning of SIBEX Sports, a titanium bike components supplier in the United States.

Acknowledgments

I want to take this opportunity to express my gratitude to the people that supported me in teaching cyclocross to our up and coming juniors over the years. The first person who thrust me into a coaching position was Jim Copeland. Jim called me one day and said that they were conducting a cyclocross camp for juniors and thought that I should be a coach. I told Jim that I don't do the coaching thing and that all I do now is the skill aspect. He quickly told me that that was perfect and I needed to show up Saturday morning at Camp Shady

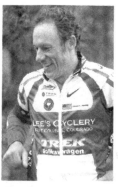

Jim Copeland

Brook in Deckers, Colorado. He wanted me there Friday night but I could not make it. So, Saturday morning I drove up and I found Jim. I approached Jim with the intention of blending into the background and just assisting the other coaches with just a few kids to teach. As soon as I found Jim, he said, "OK, You're in charge." And thus began my career as a cyclocross skill coach. Thanks, Jim (I think)!

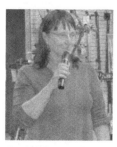

The other person I want to acknowledge is Beth-Wrenn Estes. Beth was the Executive Director for the American Cycling Association and was in charge of putting all of the cycling camps together. Beth has been an official for USAC and a UCI commissaire. She has officiated races like the Milk Race, the Olympics, the Suntour in Australia and several other national

Beth Wrenn Estes and International races. Beth has been in international cycling circles for most of her life.

Beth allowed me to be the head coach for the ACA Junior Cyclocross Camp. After a few years, we moved the camp from Deckers to Winter Park Colorado. At one point during a day at camp, I went up and said, "Beth thank you for allowing me to be the head coach here for the cyclocross camps, but I have to ask you one question."

"Sure," Beth responded.

"Why me?" I asked. "Why am I the head coach. After all I am just a no-name middle-of-the-pack guy from Oklahoma."

With a straight face she looked right at me and said, "You do what the Belgians do." When I asked what she meant by that, she pointed out that all of the drills and games that I came up with were the same as those she had seen used by the world class Belgians during her commissaire days. That was the biggest compliment that anyone has given me.

I want to also thank all of the people who helped me edit the book, Beth Wrenn-Estes, Kareena Robless, and Tim Magill.

Next, I would like to thank all of the coaches, volunteers, sponsors and parents that have given their time, energy and love to help the cyclocross camps. I am fortunate to have their help and support because without it, these camps would not be possible. Thank you.

3 Cats Photo, Beth Seliga

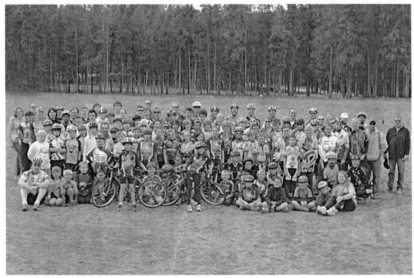

Cyclocross Campers, Staff and Volunteers

The Hard Lessons

In 1993, my mentor Randy Root really got me hooked on cyclocross. Randy would do cyclocross each winter and was good at it. From the first time I tried it I liked it. In 1994, the USCF had a cyclocross camp at the Olympic Training Center in Colorado Springs. I wanted to go; I really, really wanted to go.

I figured that the average rider would not apply because they thought they would not be able to get in. I thought that the top guys would not want to go because it would disrupt their training schedules or be subject to the politics that this sport is so well known for. In spite of all this, I applied and was accepted!

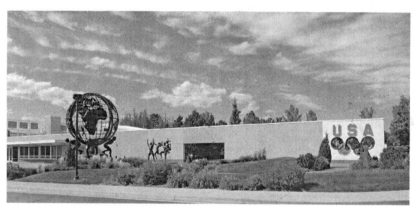

Olympic Training Center, Colorado Springs, Colorado

I arrived at the Olympic Training Center and was met by the shuttle and some of the other riders. They were from all over the US. My roommates were from California and New York. They were both better than me - A lot better than me.

Clark Natwick was the National coach at the camp. We were all brought into a meeting room for a camp meeting that night. I was about to get my first of many hard lessons. I was at the Olympic Training Center. Dreams were made there. I was high on life. Clark

got up, welcomed us to the camp, and introduced himself to us.
Clark then set the record straight as to how the USCF felt about
cyclocross. First, it was NOT an Olympic sport; therefore, it does
not receive the same support as other Olympic disciplines. Clark
told us that after camp we should head to Nationals at SeaTac. He
then told us that IF we were selected for the US team, the for
Worlds and IF we got a medal at Worlds in Switzerland we would
be compensated. Until then, the only support we would have is that
we would get some stars and bars to wear. Sure, getting a National
Team skin suit would be cool and would make a great trophy. Other
than that, we had to pay our own way. This was a shocker and my
first hard lesson. There were many more to come.

The next day Clark had us go up Ute Pass. Being from
Oklahoma I wasn't used to any type of extended climb, let alone
anything like Ute Pass. Ute Pass is a climb out of Manitou Springs
up to Woodland Park. Manitou Springs sits at about 6400 feet and
Woodland Park is close to 9300 feet above sea level. The highway
between the two is very steep and has many blind corners. The
shoulder is only two feet wide, so essentially there is no shoulder to
speak of. To me that was crazy. Apparently, it is a favorite place for
cyclists to train and all of the motorists know it, so they are aware
of the cyclists. I did not want to be hit by a car so I was the third
one to go. I figured that the more people I had behind me, the less
likely it was for me to end up as road kill. We made it to the Pikes
Peak Highway and went back. Clark made us do this twice. Some
people did it three or more times.

The next day I could barely walk. My calves were so swollen
and so sore that I had to go to medical. I went in and was met with
the standard prescription of an ice bath and a rub down. The minute
I put my legs in, I pulled them right out. It was so cold and painful
that I literally cried out. The Physical Therapist had to forcefully
hold my legs in the torture chamber of ice so that I would not pull
them out. It's a good thing the physical therapist was built like an
NFL linebacker, otherwise I would probably still be swollen and in
pain from that day.

The pain I experienced that day was worse than any race. It felt
like I had endured acupuncture administered by an epileptic with

rusty steak knives. I wanted to cry, but there were other athletes in
there from other sports and I was not going to make a sound and
bring attention to myself. The tears were flowing down my face in
buckets and I was shaking uncontrollably. Eventually I was allowed
out of the bath and taken to the massage table. I'm pretty sure the
massage therapist used a porcupine to massage my legs that day. I
suffered through biting a hand towel that they had given me. He
looked at me and said that it was okay to cry out. As much as I
wanted to cry like a little schoolgirl right then and there, I wasn't
going to let anyone see just how much this wake up call had affect-
ed me – both mentally and physically.

   The rest of the camp was just a repeat of "try and fall short"
and being reminded how bad of a cyclocross racer I really was.
Later we took a trip to Boulder to a race as a group, where only a
couple of us did well. One guy crashed into a barbed wire fence and
cut his face open. We all agreed that we would say that he got into a
knife fight.

   Clark was really mad and disappointed with every one of us. In
fact, I think everyone worked harder to get a ride back to Colorado
Springs with someone else (not
Clark) than they did in the entire
race. No one wanted to bear the
wrath of Clark on the way home.
I drew the short straw along with
three other guys. I'm pretty sure
the 90-minute drive back to the
Olympic Training Center took
eleven hours. I remember Clark
saying to me, "Well, I guess you
learned a lot today". To say that
that day was really tough for me
would be an understatement. To
some of the guys it was more like
a joy ride or a vacation while
others took it more seriously. I
took it seriously and I never for-
got it.

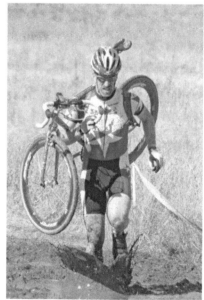

**The author taking care of
business.**

Scott Mares

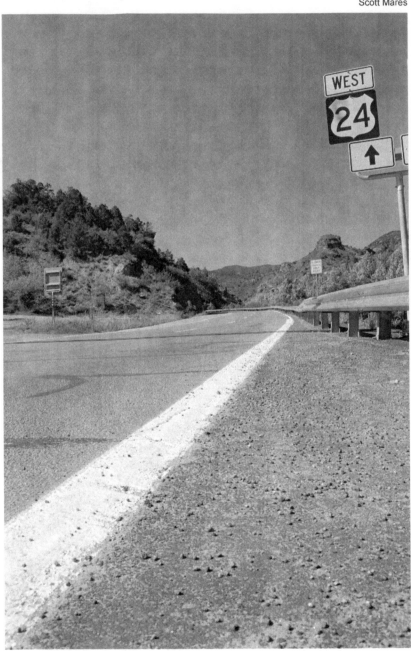

The On Ramp up Ute Pass!

Cyclocross Nationals was more of the same. I did not finish (DNF) and went home humiliated. I had a great time and I was grateful for the opportunity. I thought about the entire experience and the profound effect it had on me. I vowed that I would never be that bad ever again. When I got back home, I started to think about next year. That fall, I started to really focus on the skills needed to really excel at Cyclocross. I began to break down and analyze the movements of the dismount and remounts. I practiced this skill a half an hour before *and* after my workouts. The funny thing is, at the time I could not tell if I was getting better or if I was, by how much. The first race of the season was in Norman, OK, and I was eager to test my skill training. I raced the open and I was in the front group to the first barriers. I knew that I needed to be one of the first into the barriers. I went to the front. There were four of us that hit the barrier at the same time. After the double barriers, I had two bike lengths instantly! MONEY!

Scott Mares

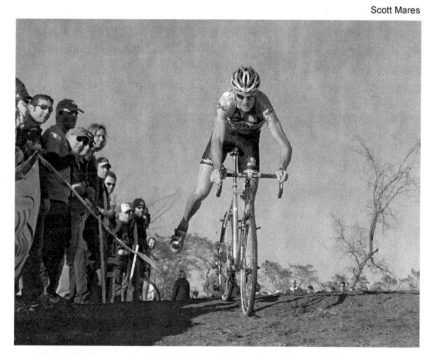

Ryan Treborn at the 2005 Crank Brothers Grand Prix.

The Purpose of This Book

Over the years, I noticed that I was being asked a lot of questions about cyclocross; and not just about basics skills. People have asked me about everything from what to wear and how to train, to tactics and what not to do. I hope that this book will answer a lot of those questions.

Later in the book, I will discuss how to train for skill. This section, will include specific details on the fastest and most efficient way to get on and off your bike. It will also include a lot of drills to hone and increase your cyclocross abilities.

In the section on race tactics, subjects will include scouting, warming up and racing. What you bring to the race is very important as well. I'll talk about what should be in your bag of tricks to help you do your best at any cyclocross race. This will include important things like clothing and key equipment.

If you want to put on a race, I can help with that too. Just like the tools that should be in your race bag, this book will give you guidance on what an ideal course should look like and where to find them. I will also cover the essentials of the race kit.

—3 Cats Photo, Beth Seliga

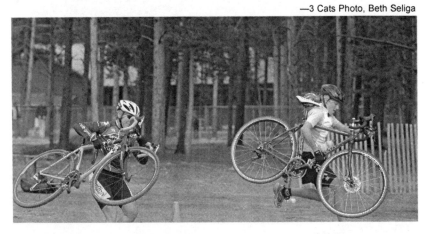

Coaches vs. riders at CX Camp at the end of drills. We set up a course just barriers and skills and race it.

Cyclocross—What Is It?

History of the Sport

Cyclocross was developed in Europe as a way for cyclists to stay fit in the winter. As the story goes, a professional cyclist wanted to train hard but could not get the resistance he needed in the mountains because of all of the snow and most of the roads being closed. This French pro had a friend that rode horseback and invited him to join him on his bike on one of his country outings. He followed his friend across the fields and over fences and up hills. He would have to get off and run

Madcross.org

with his bike. Later that summer, he won the Tour. Another story is that the cyclist would race from town to town and they were allowed to cut though the farms and did not have to adhere to the roads. The racers could take any short cut they wanted to get to the other town first. So going over fences, walls, hedges and streams was fair game. People began to take notice of this type of training and cyclocross races started popping up all over the place. It wasn't long before there was a full season dedicated to

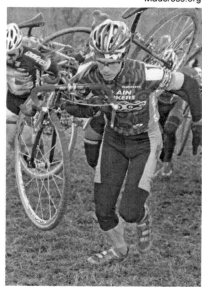
JingleCross—Iowa

this sport, complete with a World Championship. In 1954 Jean Robie won the first World Cyclocross Championships.

The Course

Cyclocross is a discipline of cycling that takes place in the fall and winter months. The course is one to three kilometers in length

with one-third of the course on a paved road and the other two-
thirds taking place off-road. The off-road portion has up to four sections with barriers 40cm tall that force the rider to dismount and run
with their bikes. The terrain is usually undulating, covered with athletic field grass. Normally the course will have a very muddy or
sandy section where the rider is forced to make a choice — run or
ride. While this is not a requirement, the spectators seem to love it.
Usually there are two pits for the riders to get either wheels or a
fresh bike. If there is only one pit, the course will go through it on
either side. This is often called a two-way pit. Generally with a two-
way pit, the course will have a figure eight shape. The pit will be
large (wide and long enough) and the bikes and wheels will be in
the center section, and the island serves as the divider of the two-
way traffic.

Cyclocross has changed over the years. The courses have
changed and thus changing the look and feel of the race. In the past,
there may have been several barrier sections and a lot of running.
This was the standard until former-pro Andre Van Der Pol was
elected in 2001 to the UCI board of cyclocross. He made changes in
the rules of cyclocross that allowed for only one barrier section.
Today, the focus of the sport is more on fitness, technical skill and
speed instead of running.

Scott Mares

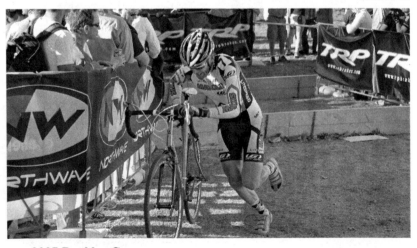

2007 Boulder Cup

The Bike

So what does a cyclocross bike look like? The typical cyclocross bike looks almost like a road bike. The main difference is that it comes with canti brakes. With closer inspection you will see that the cross bike will have skinny knobby tires and a longer wheelbase. Other than that, the bikes look like a normal road race bike. Many people will say that cross bikes have a higher bottom bracket for clearance of rocks and mud. This statement is both true and false. Back in the day (before clipless pedals), cyclocross bikes used toe clips and straps. The toe clips and straps would get caught on anything low on the ground and this could cause a rider to crash or at the least slow them down. Because of this, older cross bikes have a raised bottom bracket. Today, clipless pedals are the standard, thus eliminating the need for a higher bottom bracket on a cyclocross bike.

Scott Mares

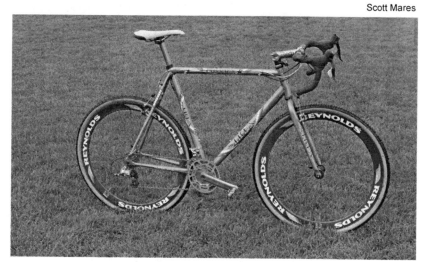

The author's bike of choice, all titanium frame and fork with deep carbon wheels.

Cyclocross Courses

Putting on a race is relatively easy to do. In fact, it is probably the easiest type of race and course to manage. The best place to host this kind of race is at city or other public parks. Multi-use parks are generally a good place because the park managers are used to the grass being walked on and know how to manage wear and tear of the area. Generally, parks that have athletic field grass are best for withstanding the wear and tear similar to that from cyclocross racing. You also need to take into consideration the available facilities. Normally parks will have a variety of accommodations that are conducive to putting on a cyclocross race, such as water, trashcans, parking and restrooms. You might even be lucky enough to have water hook ups and hoses for a bike wash.

Scott Mares

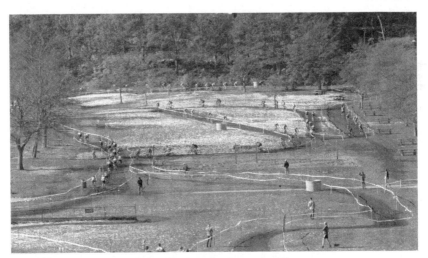

2005 U.S. Grand Prix. Notice the layout of the course.

Anatomy of the Course

The UCI rule is that the course is 2.5 to 3 kilometers in length and at least 3 meters wide throughout. Ideally, a cyclocross course should be long enough to allow for six to eight-minute laps. The best courses will snake back upon themselves and have several 180-degree turns in them. This way, you will have space for one or two pits and the racers can access them from either side of the course. The course should be wide enough to allow passing at most any point of the course. Off-camber turns, sand and undulating terrain are essential for challenging riders. The course should highlight a balance of skill and fitness. To get the greatest benfit from the course, avoid creating courses that work well with your own strengths.

The Start

The start of the course should be like an on-ramp. The start should be a separate road that feeds into the main course. The course should include a long stretch that will allow the field to string out enough so there is not a bottleneck on the course. The starting line should be marked in a grid with lanes. The grid is simply a box with lines that run parallel with the course.

Scott Mares

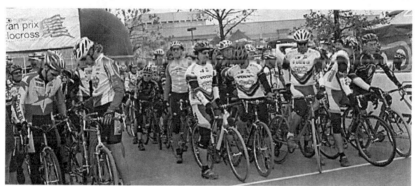

2006 U.S. Grand Prix Start Line.

The Pits

The pits should be located in the middle of the course. Ideally, you should have one large pit that can be accessed from two sides of the course. This makes it easier for every one since the riders can get a bike or a wheel from either side of the course. You will not have to have bikes and wheels in two pits at different locations, so you will only need one official in the pits to oversee it all.

Scott Mares

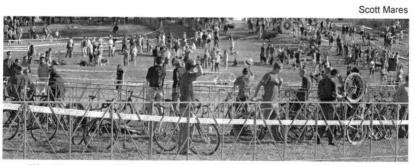

The pits at the 2007 Boulder Cup.

The Finish

The finish area should also include a long straightaway. This will make it safer if there is a sprint finish. Officials will appreciate it as well, since they will be able to see and score the race properly. Having an elevated platform for the officials to score the race would also be beneficial.

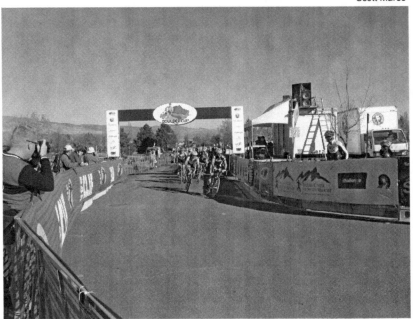

A long run into the finsh line with room afterwards.

The Course

The trick in putting together a cross course is ensuring balance. Most courses achieve this by following the one-third pavement and two-thirds off-road rule. Ideally, the off-road section is athletic field grass with undulating terrain that is at least two meters wide at every part of the course. This allows for passing and eliminates most bottlenecks. Although there is no standard for course shape, the figure eight is probably the best to start with. The figure eight shape allows for a single pit in the center and makes watching and officiating much easier for officials and spectators.

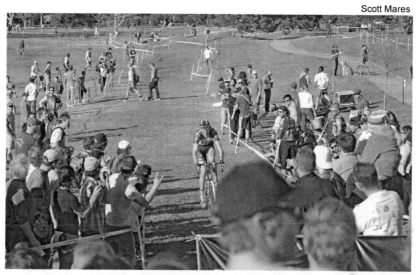

2007 Boulder Cup. Ryan Treborn off the front. Way off the front. Wide courses allow passing almost anywhere.

Once you have the basic shape to the course, you can start adding small sections onto the course. This is similar to building a house and then adding on a sidewalk, landscaping and a playground. The house is the figure eight of a cyclocross course. The sidewalks and driveways are the small sections that you add on to the course, such as pit and the start. The landscaping would be the barriers and sandy sections. These elements are considered the finishing touches to the course.

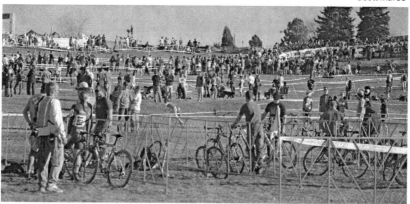

2007 Boulder Super Cup Course..

One Minute Gain

If I told you that you could gain one minute in a race with the same engine and a little skill practice you would probably think I was crazy. Well, this next section will show you how to do just that.

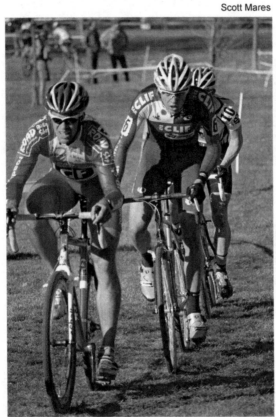
Scott Mares

2007 Boulder Cup. Riders turn it on.

Let's say you have an identical twin with an identical VO_2 max (aerobic capacity) and LT (Lactate Threshold). You go to a cyclocross skill camp, but your twin does not. When you are there, you learn how to get on and off your bike efficiently and you continue to practice on a weekly basis after camp is over. Now let's say that all that hard work and practice has gotten you only one second faster though the barriers than your identical twin. If the race is ten laps long and has four barrier sections, after five laps you would be 20 seconds ahead of your twin. If we take into account fatigue and some mistakes your twin will make during the latter half of the race, you are probably now two seconds faster through the barriers than your twin. So, if my calculations are correct (and they should be after going through the first grade twice), in the final five laps you gain 40 seconds in addition to the 20 seconds you gained in the first half of the race. This means you would beat your identical twin by one whole minute. Go back through the results of your previous cyclocross races and see how close you were to your competition at the end. After some correct practice, you should be close to closing that margin on your competition.

Being efficient on and off the bike can make a vast difference over the course of a race. A rider that is trying to stay with you though the barriers will most likely lose time or crash if they are not as efficient in dismounting and remounting as you are. That pressure will cause them to make a mistake and lose large amounts of time. If they back off, they will have to make extra efforts to catch back up to you, which will most likely result in them blowing up too soon. Smooth, controlled and efficient techniques will allow you put all of your energy into going forward.

Scott Mares

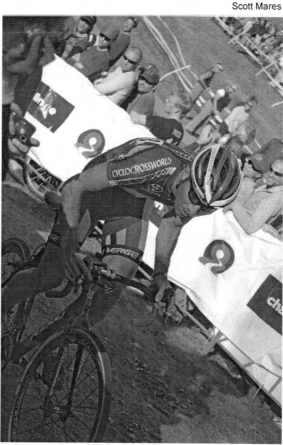

2007 Boulder Cup. J. Powers turns it on.

The Three Keys to Cyclocross

This section is the foundation of your skill training for cyclocross. If you do these three movements in order, you will go faster than you have before in a cyclocross race. Scramble the order of these three key moves or leave one out and I guarantee you will either lose time or crash. I have put the three movements into an easy to understand and simple catchphrase: Scissor, Top-tube, Barrier. This is the key to cyclocross. You need to say this 10 times a day and make it second nature.

So what does it mean? Each word stands for the movement in getting off the bike. I will say it again: **IF YOU DO THIS OUT OF SEQUENCE OR FAIL TO DO ANY OF THEM, YOU WILL EITHER LOSE TIME OR CRASH.** So, it's *very* important that you learn each step in order.

Scissor

The scissor movement starts simply by un-clicking your right foot out of your pedal and bringing it back behind your saddle fol-

J. Patrick Bernard

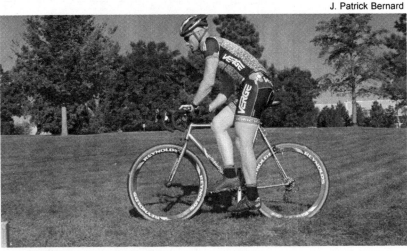

The Scissor Position. Note that the right leg is forward of the left leg and the toe is pointed down in prep for the foot strike. Strike with the toe and not the heel.

lowed by moving your right leg up between your left leg and your frame. Then you will move your right leg forward and bend your right knee. Your right knee is "cocked" like the hammer on a gun and your toe should be pointed down slightly. This will be the leg that strikes the ground first when you dismount at speed. Your hands can be either on the tops of the bars or on the drops. This will depend largely on the situation. For most situations, the tops are the best choice.

Top-Tube

When you have finished the scissor movement, you are now free to execute the top tube movement. This will allow you to stay in control of your bike and keep your balance when you dismount. With your RIGHT hand, release the handlebar and move your hand across the top of the handle bar until you find your stem (don't look, feel your way). Keep going from your stem to your top tube and then loosely conform your hand around it and slide it all the way back until your forearm hits the nose of the saddle. This is very important because this is where you are going to pick the bike up. If you don't go all the way back to the nose of the saddle, when you pick your bike up it will be un-balanced and the bike will nose up.

J. Patrick Bernard

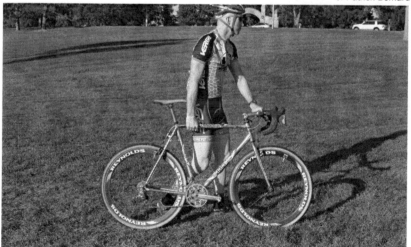

Correct grab of the top tube of the bike.

This will cause you to hit the back wheel on the barrier. Hitting the barrier with your bike at speed can cause you to lose control of your bike. This could also damage your bike or cause you to crash. Both are undesirable situations in cyclocross. With one hand at the front and one at the back, when you pick up the bike it will be balanced.

J. Patrick Bernard

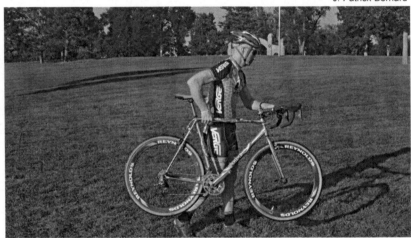

Bike is lifted evenly.

J. Patrick Bernard

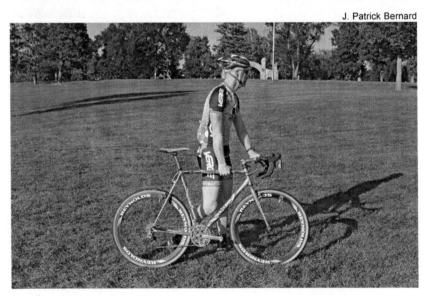

WRONG place to grab the top tube. The hand is too far forward.

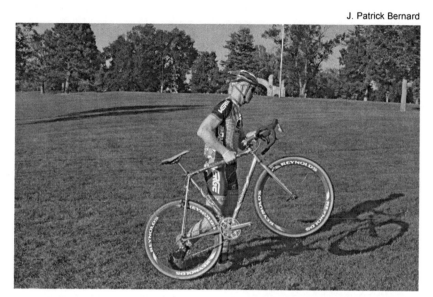

This is why it is WRONG. The bike is unbalanced, the front end is up, and the rear wheel is dragging and will hit something.

Barrier

This is the final stage in this sequence. Barrier is the actual execution of going over the barrier. In this sequence, you will click out of your left pedal, step through with your right leg and start running. As your take the barrier, pick the bike up with both hands and lift it up and over the barrier. When you lift the bike to go over a barrier or obstacle, lift it evenly keeping it parallel to the ground. When you watch other people go over the barrier, note how high they lift the bike up. You should lift it just enough to clear the barrier. Anything beyond that is a waste of energy. When you sit the bike back on the ground you want to let it down easily. As you are putting the bike down, thrust the bike slightly in front of you as if you were releasing a bowling ball. **DO NOT DROP THE BIKE.** Dropping the bike can cause you to drop your chain, mess your wheel up or damage your bike in some other manner.

J Pastore Bernard

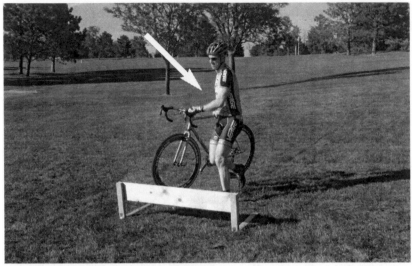

Note hands on bar and top tube.

J Pastore Bernard

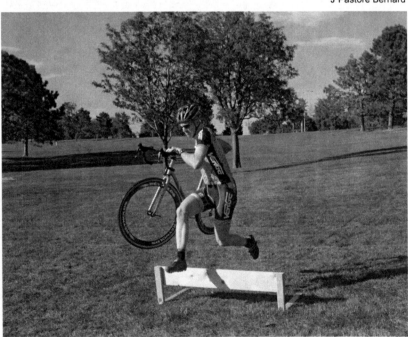

Bike is level and in control.

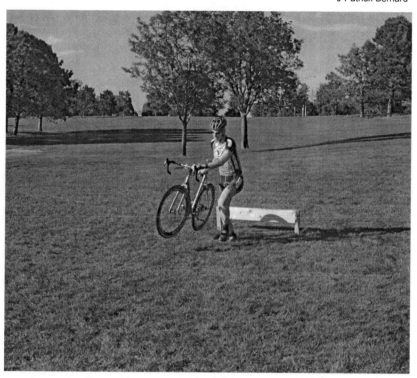

Over the barrier and starting the landing.

The Flick

This is a move used by many top pros when you need to get over a barrier but don't need or want to lift the bike all the way up. It is also used if you are changing directions and immediately going over a barrier. So what is the Flick? When executing the flick, you don't lift the bike. Instead, you flick it sideways as you go over a barrier. The wheels go out and away from you. Now, you do have to pick the bike up a little bit just not the entire 41cm. In the movement, you push the left part of the handlebars down and twist the top tube in towards you. This will cause the bike to pitch sideways. After you clear the barrier, bring the bike vertical again and proceed.

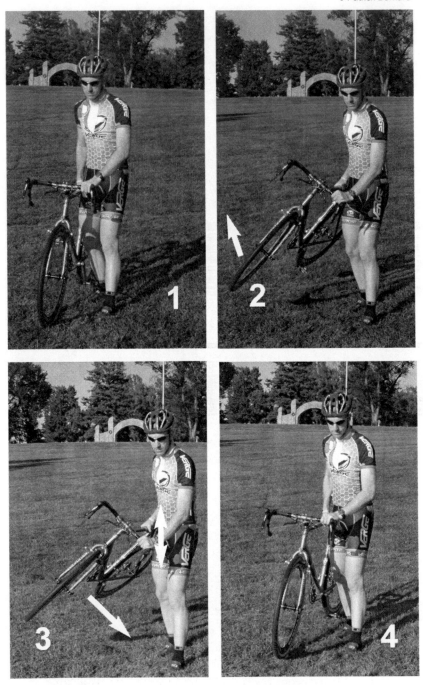

The author demonstrating the flick in sequence.

Cowboy Dismount

If you are going to have to dismount at a point that makes you lose all of your momentum and you don't have time to step through, or you are going to dismount with a change in direction (a right turn), then the "Cowboy Dismount" is the way to go. This is simply done not by stepping through but by stepping behind. Also you have the option of keeping your hands on the bars or having one on the top tube. The reason it's called the "Cowboy Dismount" is this is how the cowboys get off their horses in a hurry. You will see them doing this in all of the westerns where the hero rushes into town and gets off his horse before it has totally stopped.

Shouldering the Bike

There will come a time when you will need to shoulder the bike. There are a handful of situations when shouldering the bike is the only way to go. In most cases, it is largely dependent on the person and their running technique. You will have to figure out which way is faster or more energy efficient for you by experimenting (i.e. trial and error). Now, there are several types of situations (coming into a barrier section) when you can choose to shoulder. Again, this is highly dependent on the course; each one is different. Generally speaking, there are two scenarios where you should shoulder the bike. The first one is the high-speed straight-on dismount. The other includes situations like non-straight-on approach, off-camber, right angle, or rough dismounts. In each instance, you are going to have to shoulder the bike. The technique however, will vary.

First, let's talk about the standard high-speed shoulder sequence. Earlier we laid the foundation with the "Scissor – Top Tube – Barrier" approach. When shouldering the bike, the sequence becomes, "Scissor – Down Tube – Barrier." As you might have guessed, the only change is that you grab the down tube instead of the top tube.

The execution is the same. As you click-out of your left pedal and step through with your right foot, pull up the down tube and push down with the left hand (hands on the tops of the bar). This will

J. Patrick Bernard

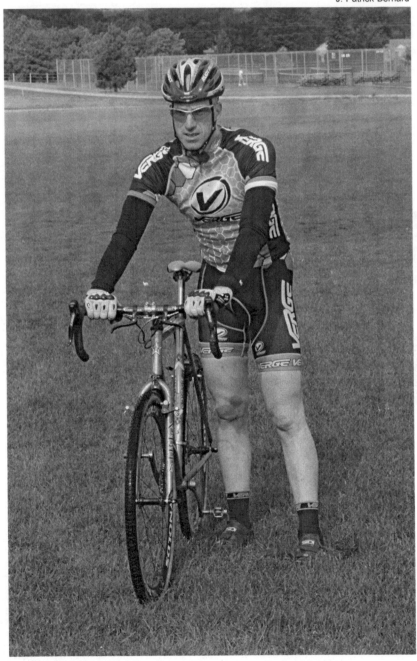

The starting position. Both hands on the top of the bar.

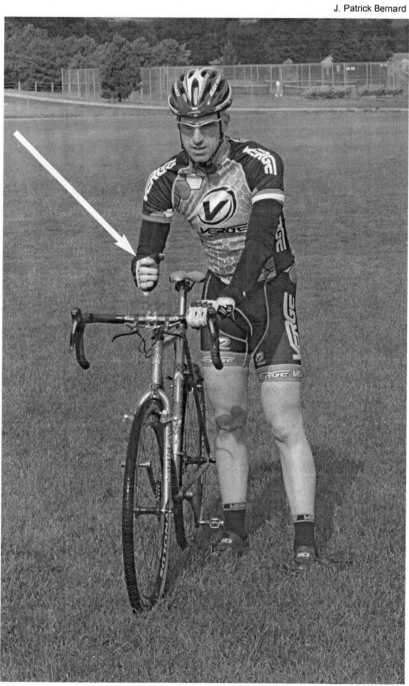

Right hand is off the bar and going to the top tube.

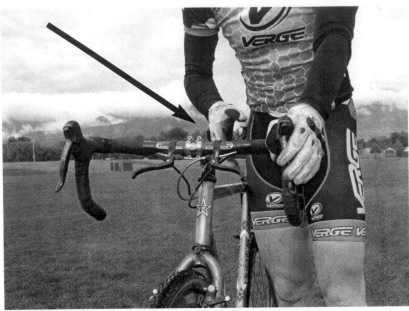

Hand is getting ready to go straight down.

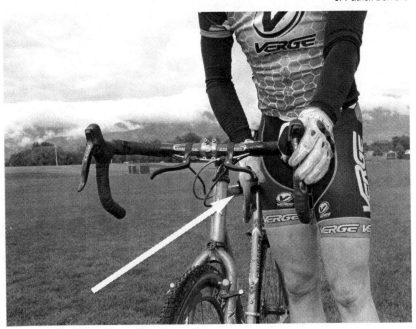

Hand is flat and heading straight down.

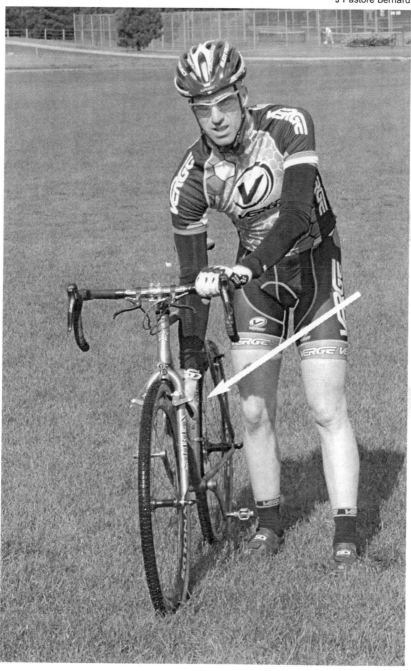

Hand has gripped the down tube.

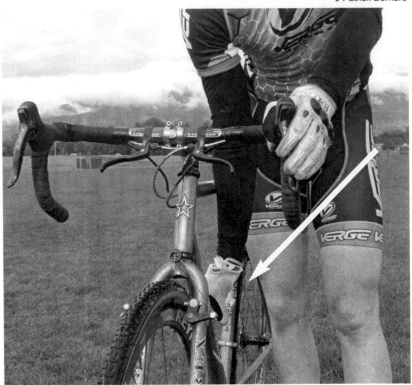

Close-up of the grab of the down tube.

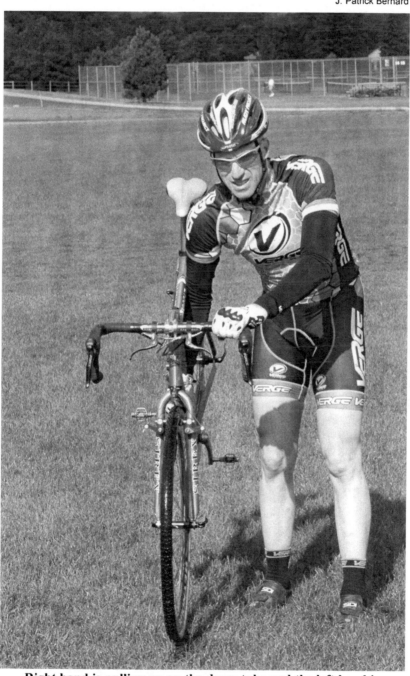

Right hand is pulling up on the down tube and the left hand is pushing forward. The rear wheel is coming up.

J. Patrick Bernard

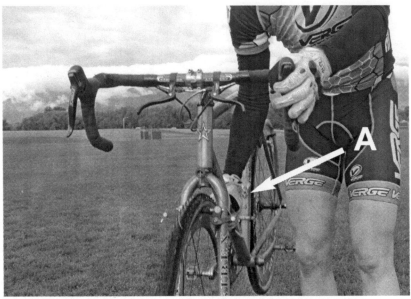

Start of bike being lifted up. (A) Right hand on down tube.

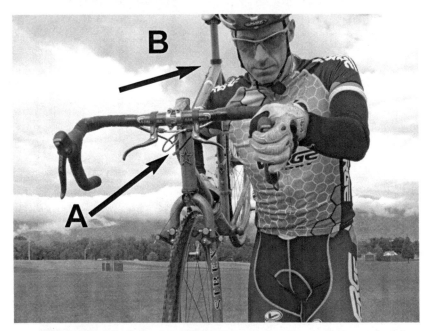

**Bike being lifted up. (A) Right elbow going through the main tri-
angle and (B) bike going on the shoulder.**

J. Patrick Bernard

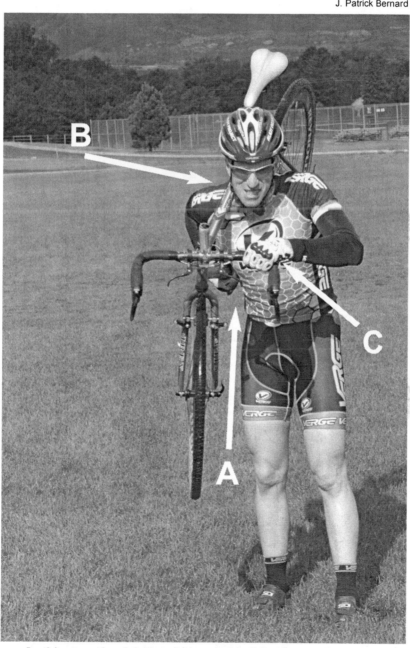

In this step, the right hand has a hold of the down tube (A) and has brought the frame up and on to the shoulder (B). The left hand is still on the top of the bars (C).

J. Patrick Bernard

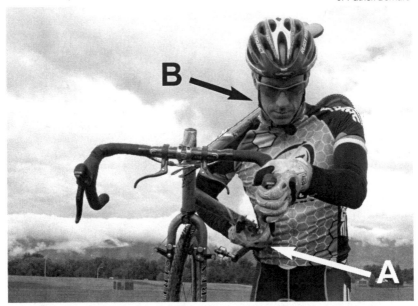

(A) The right hand has released the down tube and is going for the end of the handle bar. (B) The bike is on the shoulder.

J. Patrick Bernard

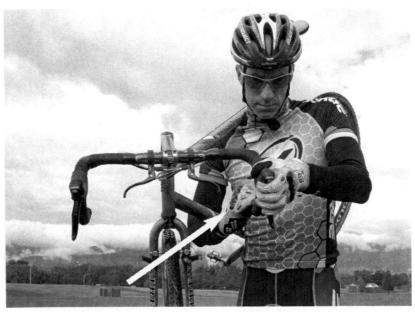

The right hand has grabbed the end of the handle bar.

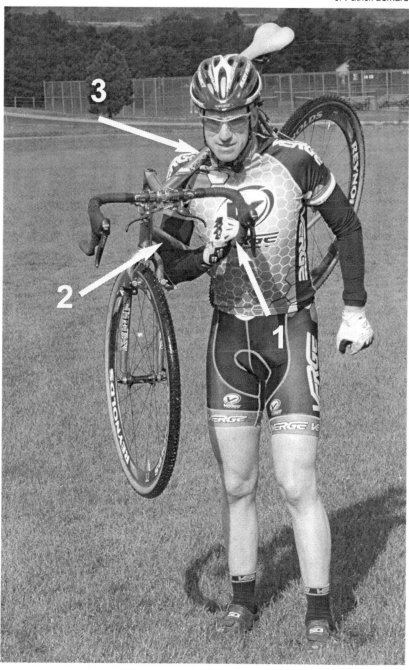

The three points of contact. This will give you more control over
over you bike while running.

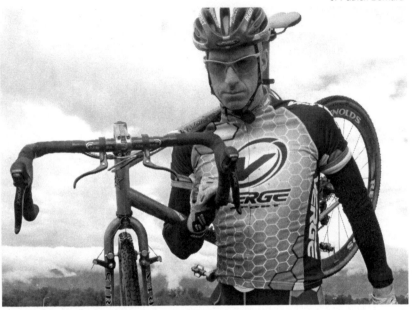

Closer view of the three points of contact.

J. Patrick Bernard

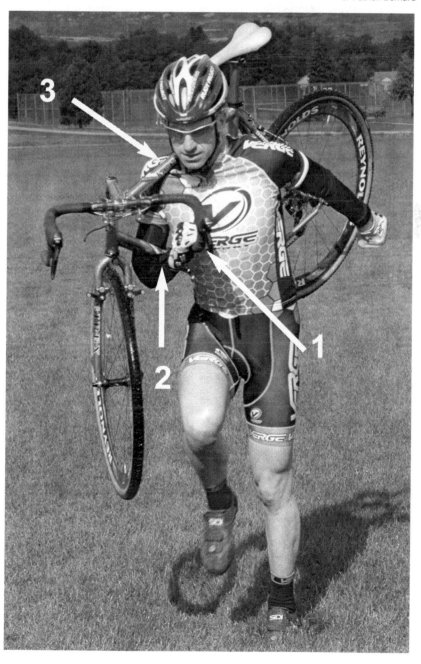

What it looks like while running.

cause the rear of the bike to kick up and the nose of the bike to stay down. The pivot of the bike in this movement is the head tube. As you are doing this, your right elbow kicks out through the main triangle of the frame. At this point, open your right hand from the down tube and reach for the opposite handle bar end (left) with your right hand. When you do this, your forearm will be under and supporting the down tube. The middle of the top tube will be on your shoulder at this point. This is the most stable way to run with the bike because you now have three contact points in which to hold the bike. This way, the weight of the bike is not just concentrated in one spot.

Your three contact points are (1) the right hand on the end of the handle bar, (2) the down tube resting on your right forearm and (3) the center of the top tube on your shoulder. So where do you place the bike on your shoulder? The best spot to shoulder your bike is on the shoulder neck junction. Make sure you place it on the muscle part of your shoulder, not a spot where there is bone.

After you have successfully shouldered the bike, run to the top of the run up. To place the bike back on the ground, follow these three steps. Like in "Scissor – Down Tube – Barrier," there are also three steps in this movement:

■   Step 1 - Take your left hand and place it on the top of the handle bar.

■   Step 2 - Release your right hand from the handle bar and make a hook with your hand. Straighten out your right arm and let the bike slide off your shoulder and down your arm. Catch the down tube with your right hand.

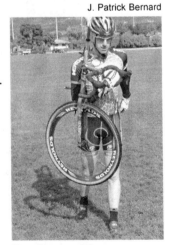

J. Patrick Bernard

■   Step 3 - Put the bike on the ground. Now the trick is to put the bike down gently. **DO NOT DROP THE BIKE!** Use the same bowling action as before to put the bike on the ground. This will also start the bike moving forward.

Starting position.

J. Patrick Bernard

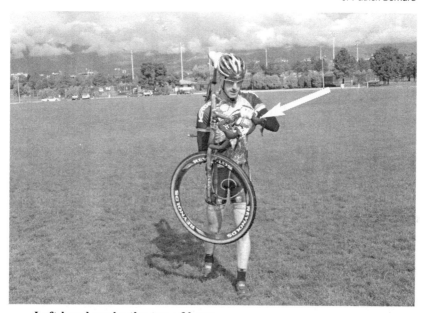

Left hand grabs the top of bars.

J. Patrick Bernard

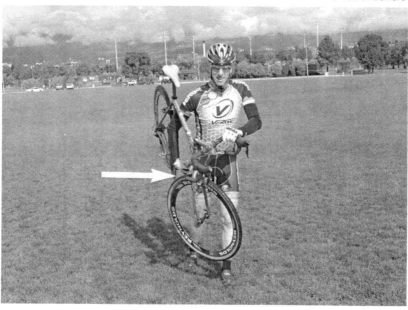

Right hand releases bar end and grabs the down tube. Frame comes off the shoulder.

J. Patrick Bernard

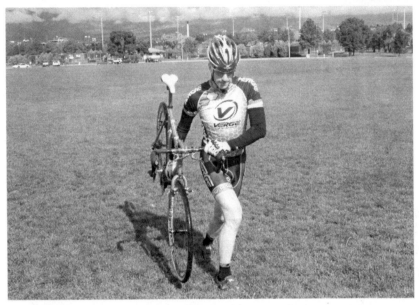

Bike is now in the approach (process of landing).

J. Patrick Bernard

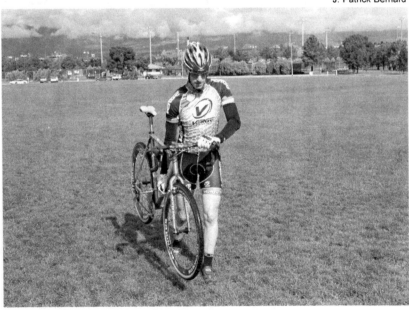

Leveling out for the landing.

J. Patrick Bernard

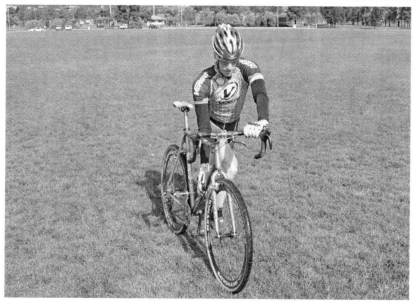

Bike had landed and is "bowled forward." Right hand is releasing.

J. Patrick Bernard

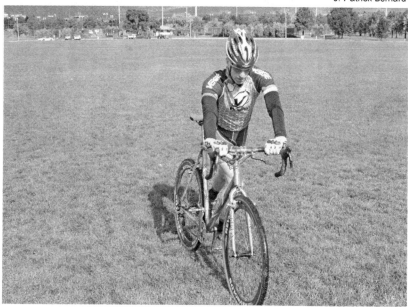

Right hand is now on the top of the bars and ready for removal.

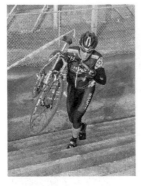

Sun Prairie, Wisconsin, Angeell Park Speedway Cyclocross. Angle run with stairs.

Let's talk about the non-standard unstable shoulder technique. This technique is used when the dismount is not straight-on with a smooth approach; it's off-camber; or something about it is making the approach difficult or unstable. Each situation is going to be different. The rougher the approach, the longer you have to stay mounted with a slower speed. The other factor is the change of direction for the run-up. Many promoters like to make the run-up at a 90-degree angle from the approach. What this means is that when you are on the approach, you have to dismount and then change directions by 90 degrees and do a run up. This increases the level of difficulty because all of your momentum is going in the direction of the approach and then you have to change directions.

Because of the change of direction, it is better to grab the top tube of the bike, pull the frame up, grab the down tube of the frame and shoulder the bike to run the section. The other option is to dismount and shoulder the bike before the change of direction in the run-up section. You will have to experiment to find out which way is more comfortable for you and works best with your strengths.

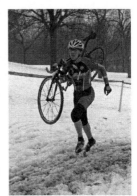

2007 Wisconsin State Cyclocross Championship

Now there is another reason to shoulder a bike. I was in a race in Morrison, Colorado and there was a very steep ditch in the run-down area, it was too short to ride down and dismount to come up the other side. The other side of the ditch had stairs carved out of the side of it. The route of this section was down and then a hard 90-degree left to the other side. There was quite a bit of ice on the course as well. In this situation, it was faster to shoulder the bike and run through the ditch instead of trying to make correction while on the bike.

Inga Wortman

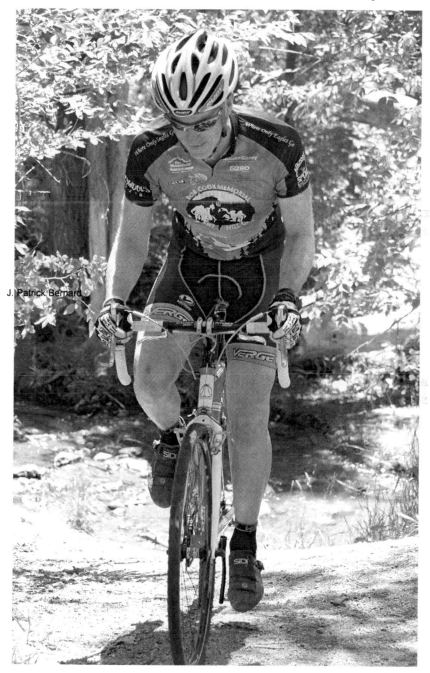

J. Patrick Bernard

The Remount

In this section, we will talk about remounting without causing major damage to your saddle area. Contrary to popular belief, this is just as important for men as it is for women. After you have successfully gone over the barrier and placed the bike back on the ground, accelerate up to speed (running). When you leap back on, your right inner thigh should be the first thing to land on the saddle. Once your thigh has made contact, slide it down the curve of the saddle. The curve is the part from the nose to the flair where you sit. DO NOT land on your butt (or anything else for that matter). Once you are back in the saddle; extend your legs to the pedals, engage your cleats and start pedaling.

When you execute this movement, your leg should follow an arc shape onto the saddle. I would say that the movement is similar to putting your arm around your loved one or best friend. This arc should only go a little bit higher than the saddle. Your inner thigh

J. Patrick Bernard

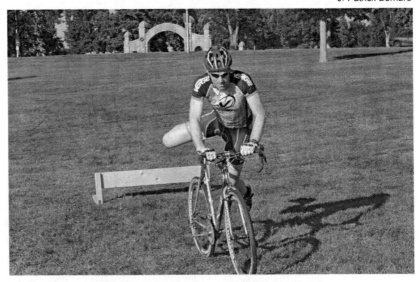

Notice the inner thigh is just above the saddle.

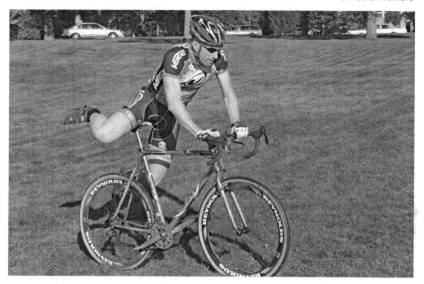

The inner thigh is sliding onto the saddle...

should hit the saddle at a descending angle. The part of the saddle that you want to shoot for is the outside curve. This curve is where the nose of the saddle flares out to the large part of the saddle. Your thigh should slide through the center of this curve down to the pedals using the curve as a guide for your thigh

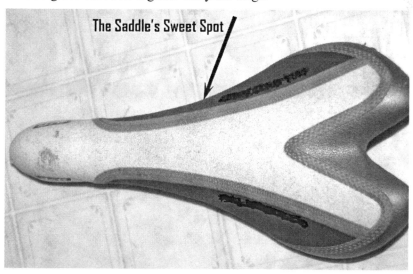

The Saddle's Sweet Spot

Do not jump onto the saddle. Jumping up and landing directly on the saddle is not a good thing. I'm actually going to call that...BAD. Jumping high and landing on the saddle will put a tremendous amount of stress on the seat post and could cause it to break. I have seen this happen several times. Not only will this ruin your race, it could ruin your weekend (if you know what I mean).

This remounting movement is very similar to that of the trail leg for a hurdler. Stand next to your bike on the non-drive side and place your right knee on the center of the saddle. Once you do this, the similarities of the movement should be obvious. This position is actually a good stretch for your body and a way to get use to the idea of getting on the bike. It will also help in your body's spatial awareness for getting on the bike

Skill Drills

In this section, I will cover the drills that you need to do over and over again. The drills themselves are not physically tough, but they are tough mentally because of the number of repetitions. However, the rewards you will gain will be very noticeable.

I want you to have two concepts: that the individual skill drills are progressive and modular. This means that you can take any individual drill and make them harder (progressive) and put them together (modular) to form a series of drills. However, you need to be experienced in doing the individual drills and their progressions first before you do them in a series or in sucession. This also means that when you start your skill training session you should start with the basics and progress to more difficult drills. Getting your body warm and use to the ballistic movements is key to correct training. If you don't you will not maximize the training and you could also injure yourself.

Where to Do Skill Drills

You want to find a place that has plenty of room and a lot of flat smooth ground. The best places are city parks. The grass tends to be athletic field grass and there is usually plenty of room to do drills. If they have some rollers in them even better! The other great thing about parks is that usually you will live pretty close to one so it's not too far of a ride or drive. Everyone knows where they are and you can have a group meet up there and have practice. Another thing great about parks is if you fall it won't hurt as much if you fell on a big rock or tree stump/log.

On and Off

This is the most basic and the most important drill. Because it's so basic and used all the time, it must be mastered to the point that it becomes second nature to the cyclocross racer. To do this drill, find a large, flat grassy area in a park. Before doing this drill, make sure your muscles are warmed up. Spend 30 minutes getting on and off the bike. This drill includes clipping into AND out of your pedals. After you have done 30 min of this drill, go and do the rest of your normal work out. When you are done with your workout, come back and do another 30 minutes of this same drill. Keep in mind, this skill must be mastered and reinforced, especially when you are tired. Common sense dictates that in the race, you will get tired and your form will suffer. This is when most mistakes are made and the most time is lost. They are generally costly mistakes and hard to recover from.

Shoulder On and Off

In this drill, you will be shouldering the bike just as you would during the running section of a cyclocross course. Begin with the classic "Scissor – Top Tube – Barrier" sequence, but instead of putting your hand on the top tube, grab the down tube. When you take your right hand off the brake lever, move your hand towards the top tube with your palm facing away from the tube. The back of your hand will slide against the side of the top tube as you reach straight down. Your hand should make contact with the down tube right above the bottle mounts. Now, use your left hand to push down on the handlebars as you pull up with your right hand. This will cause the bike to pivot nose down and bring the rear up allowing you to place the top tube on your shoulder. Your right arm

3 Cats Photo, Seliga

Haulman demonstrates scissors weave drill at CX camp.

then goes under the down tube and reaches up to grab the left end of the handlebars. This will turn the handlebars and prevent the arm from being wedged between the frame and the wheel. This hold gives you three contact points and because you have total control of the bike, it won't flail around. You must practice this drill until it becomes second nature to you if you are to do it in a race at high speed. If you do, others will not be able to match the move and a gap will instantly open up. If you make a mistake, it will be costly, in both time and energy, so spend the time and master this skill.

Weave Drills

This is a drill in which you will need several cones to set up in a line. The objective is to increase quick handling skills for maneuvering in tight areas. Set the cones up in a line with approximately three to four bike lengths between each. Ride towards the line of cones and weave in and out of them. The first pass should be taken somewhat easy and with each additional pass increase the speed. After several times through the cones, repeat the drill and decrease the space between the cones. Try to go through the cones as fast as possible. Be creative in your set up. Set up your cones on a hill or hillside (off-camber), rough terrain or in a crooked line. This drill can also be done as a group, making a game out of it.

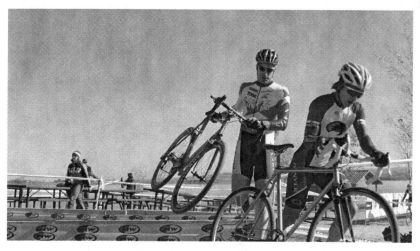

The author taking double barriers in Colorado.

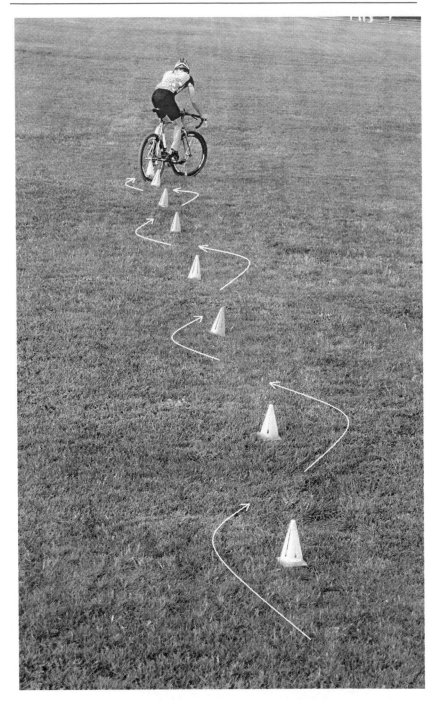

Weave drill example

Single Barrier

This drill should only be done after you have mastered the on-and-off and can dismount correctly. Truth be told, it's not that hard to get on and off the bike when you have nothing coming at you. However, obstacles such as barriers and steps force you to re-calculate your pedal stroke, gear and braking tactics. This is where most mistakes are made and the field is separated. If you can get off and on your bike as easily as you tie your shoe (I'm taking a chance and assuming that tying your shoe is second nature) then you should have no problem with a single barrier. Placement of the barrier is critical. Place the barrier on flat level ground. After you master the single barrier, change the position of the barrier. Place it on rough or off-camber ground. Placing it right after a 180-degree turn is another good skill to try. Try to think of real race situations where promoters place barriers. A slight incline or at the top of a hill is a common race element. The things that you want to look for are how close you get to the barrier. How many steps do you take before going over the barrier? Ideally, you should be taking two steps before you cross the barrier—three is too many and one is not enough. If you only take one step, you will most likely crash because one step will not provide you enough stability at speed to control yourself. If you find yourself taking three steps, try to get

J. Patrick Bernard

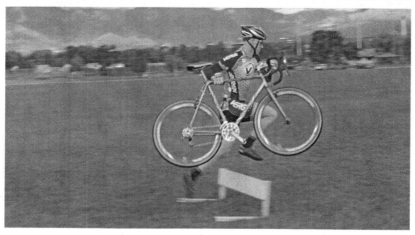

The author takes a single barrier at speed.

closer until you can comfortably do it in two.

If you are still struggling to get your dismount down to two steps, try this tip. Take something to mark where another rider (one who is able to do it in two steps) gets off. Place the marker where his foot first hits the ground, use that marker as a target for you. **Do not do this at full speed.** This should be done at half speed so you will feel more in-control and not feel rushed in the movement. If this doesn't work, slowly ride into the barrier to hit it and knock over the barrier. You need to understand that the barrier will fall over and if you hit the barrier you will not crash. In doing this exercise it will show you that the risk of crashing is actually very small.

Double Barrier

This is the same drill as the single barrier only with two barriers. Once again, you need to master the on-and-off before starting barrier drills. For two barriers, experiment with the distance between the two. Start out with the barriers two-bike lengths apart. After a couple of passes, put more distance between them until you get to the point where you could either run between the two or remount. This will challenge you in your decision-making skills concerning running or remounting and riding. After this, place the barriers on varied terrain as in the single barrier drill.

Placing double barriers on a hill or off-camber are excellent places to test and improve your skills. Placing them in rough terrain, mud or sand will add another dimension to the drill. You can be as creative as you want, however try to mimic those elements that you will most likely find in a race.

Turning, 90,180, and 360

Typically, when we go out and train we don't do any training for turning. It's only in the race that we encounter 180 turns. Practicing this drill will pay off greatly in a race. Find a park with some trees in it. Ride to the tree and ride a tight circle around it. Ride to the next tree and turn in the opposite direction. Keep trying to turn as tight as possible and as quickly as possible. If you can find two trees close together, do a figure eight drill in each direction. This skill drill will force you to not only to turn your bike, but it will make use your entire body in the turn.

Cone Racing

This is a fun drill to do if you have at least one other person to race against and in all it is a great fitness equalizer. Your big turbo engine is not that helpful here, so riders of all levels of abilities can do this together. For this drill, you need at least three cones and at least two people; three to four people are ideal, but this depends on the course. The larger the course, the more people you can have. The purpose of this drill is to demonstrate that it is not always the first person to the cone who wins.

Take three cones and set them up in a triangle. They should be wide enough apart that you can take two pedal strokes between the cones (3-5 bike lengths apart should be good). This drill is a race where everyone begins *off* their bikes. Have everyone line up 30 meters from the center of the triangle. After the signal to start has been given, riders race to the far cone on the left or right side. Complete an inside-out circle of the first and second cones. The last cone is an outside-in circle followed by a race back to the start. This exercise will make you more aware of placement, lines, braking, gears and speed. You can mix up the order of the cones (pattern) that you do or the number of cones that you have. Make sure that everyone knows the pattern before the start of the race.

Bunny Hops

Although this may seem like a simple drill, it is a necessary skill to have in cyclocross. The purpose of this drill is to increase your ability to hop obstacles and maintain control of your bike. Just roll up and hop, bringing the entire bike with you. Both tires should come off the ground at the same time. Do three hops then roll out and back, adding two more hops each time. After you have mastered this skill, get a board or a dowel. Paint it white and it will be easier for you to focus on the task. Roll up parallel to the dowel, stop and bunny hop to the other side of the dowel, and then roll through. Do this until you have mastered going over it. The next time through, start from the opposite side and perform this task the other way. After you are comfortable with this task, roll up and bunny hop from one side to the other over the dowel. Try this multiple times.

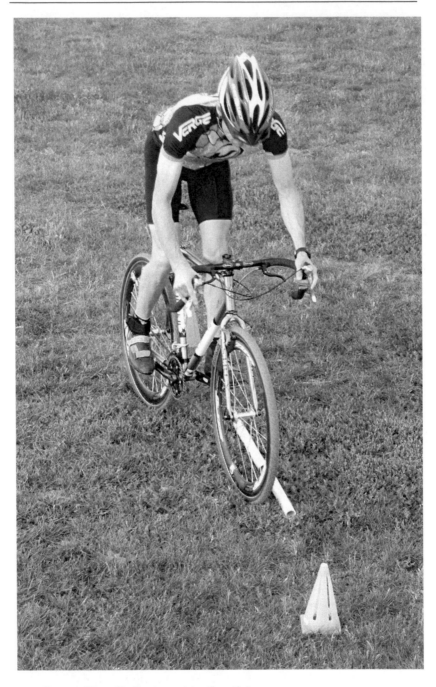

Bunny Hop: Roll up next to the stick.

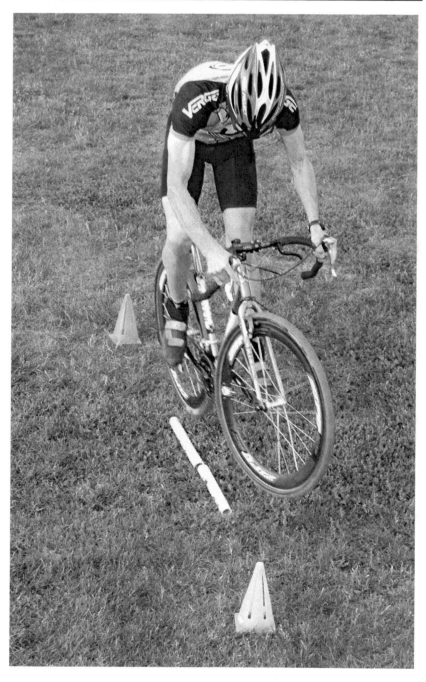

Bunny Hop: In mid-hop, and directly over the stick.

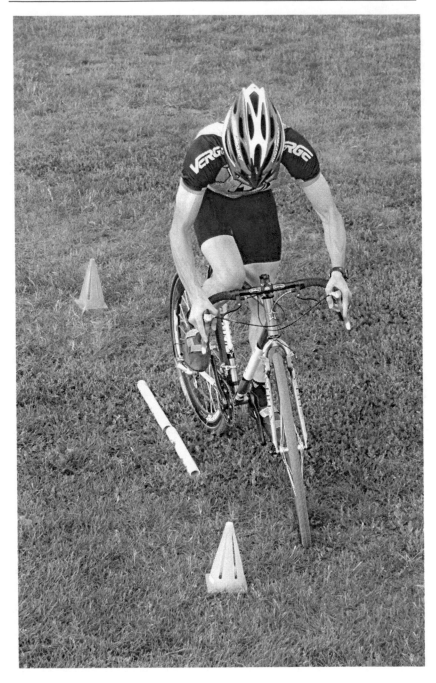

Bunny Hop: The landing. Safely on the other side.

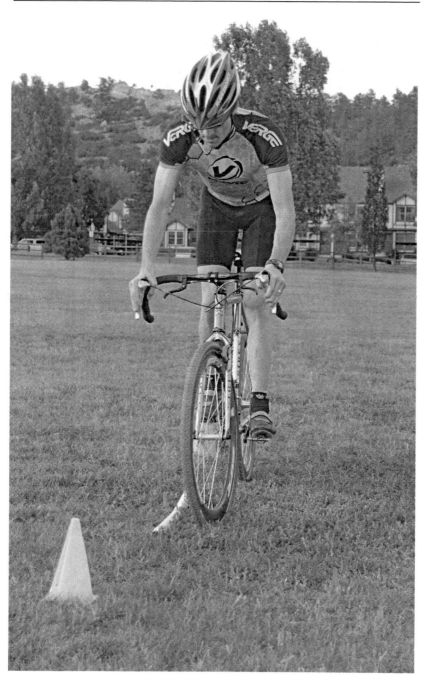

Bunny Hop: Roll up next to the stick.

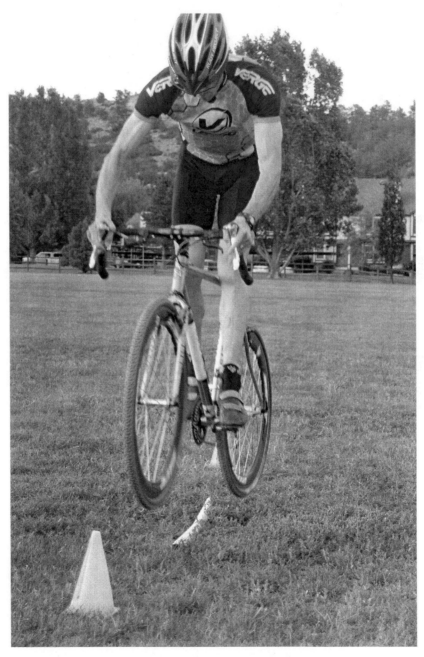

Bunny Hop: In mid-hop, and directly over the stick.

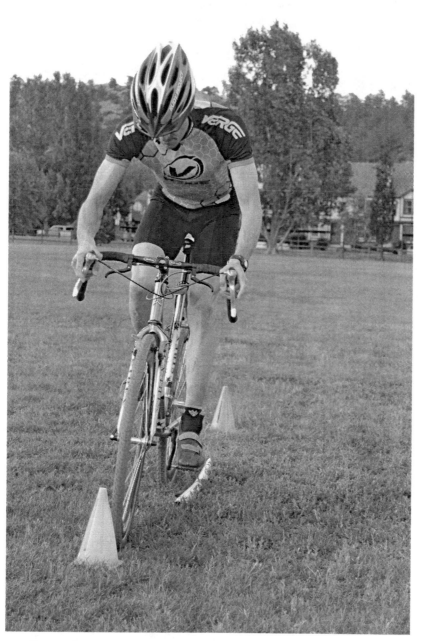

Bunny Hop: The landing. Safely on the other side.

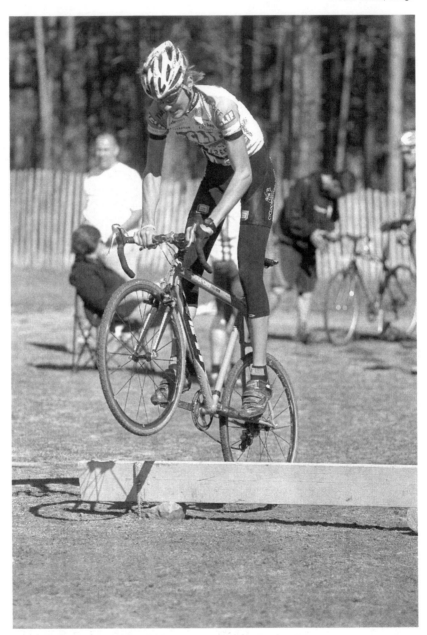

Kappis bunny-hopping barrier at CX Camp.

Scissor Riding

This exercise will increase your comfort, stability and control in the scissor position. To do this, find a flat smooth piece of park space. Accelerate your bike and get some speed because you are going to coast. After reaching your speed, go into the scissor position and hold it. Both hands should be on the hoods or tops of the bars. Your right hip should be resting against the saddle. Your right leg should be in the scissor position and bent with the toe pointed down. While in this position, proceed in a straight line.

As you build your confidence, add turns and weaves into this exercise; adding some cones to weave though increases the difficulty. Try this drill going straight downhill; on the off-camber part of a hill; or try snaking back-and-forth while descending a hill.

J. Patrick Bernard

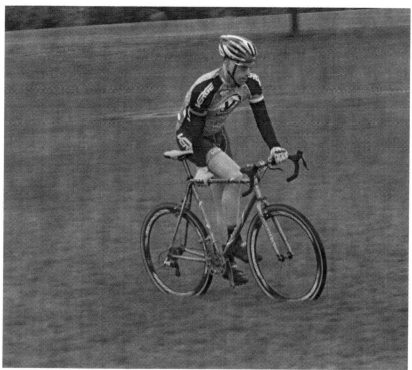

The author demonstrating scissor riding.

Wagon Wheels

This drill is a variation of the bunny hop. Mastering Wagon Wheels will increase your ability to control your bike. It will also teach you to move the rear end of the bike while continuing to move in the direction you want to go. Start by bunny hopping in-place. When you are in the air, kick the rear end of your bike out and change direction while keeping your front wheel in the same spot. Keep doing this until you have made a complete circle. Once you have mastered doing this in one direction, try it going the other way. After doing this several times, you should feel your core warming up. This is a great core workout as well!

Power Slides

One major component of cyclocross is staying in control of your bike. A rider should be able to ride right up to the edge of being out of control and know where that is and what that feels like. Test pilots put planes into a spin or stall and learn how to recover out of this situation bringing the aircraft back under their control. This is exactly what this drill will do for the rider. This drill can be done on a variety of terrains and conditions.

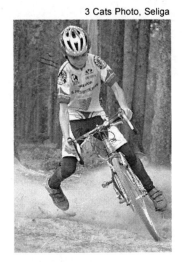

3 Cats Photo, Seliga

Start on a flat area, accelerate quickly, and lock up the rear brake. Put the bike into a rear wheel skid and fish-tail the end out to the left or right, then recover from the slide and continue riding. This exercise should be done repeatedly in both directions (left and right). Change-up the terrain so that it becomes more difficult to maintain control of the bike. Wet grass, hillsides and loose dirt all affect your ability to control your bike. I guarantee you will face all of these conditions in a race at some point.

NM CX Camper does a power slide

Running Turns.

Use a cone or a tree. Race to the cone/tree and at a particular point (Before the cone/tree) have a mandatory dismount either with or with out a barrier so you run with your bike around the cone/tree (180 degree turn) and then remount and accelerate. Easy- flat & level, change the terrain to increase the difficulty. Even make it a down hill approach to the turn so that it's a down hill run to the turn and a uphill run after the turn. Make sure you run this drill both ways. This means a left turn and then a right turn.

Track Stand

This drill will enable you to come to a complete stop without putting a foot down or falling over. One of the most important points in a race is the start and the dash to the first corner. This is called the "The Hole Shot." Often times this bottle neck in the field will cause other riders to go down. If you are caught behind this mess and you have to put a foot down, it's much harder to get going again. If you were in a track stand, then you can just punch it and leave the other riders behind.

This drill is best done on a slight uphill grade, as this will make the maneuver easier to execute. The uphill grade should be very subtle in nature. Start by rolling up to a point a few yards ahead of you. Begin to slow down to the point of stalling as you approach this point. Once you have reached the stalling point, turn the handlebars into the hill/rise/incline. At this point, apply the brakes and have your pedals in the 3 o'clock and 9 o'clock position. Allow the bike to roll backwards a few inches, and then apply just enough force to make the bike roll forward slightly. Do this again and you will notice a slight rocking motion even though you will be at a stand still. The more advanced you become, the less the rocking motion and less of an incline you will need.

Bump and Thump

The first road camp that the American Cycling Association had was in Deckers, Colorado in the springtime. Springtime in the Rocky Mountains is by definition a very soggy time. One of the

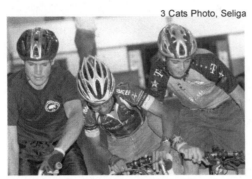

3 Cats Photo, Seliga

Three campers battle in Bump & Thump.

rainy day activities we had the kids do was the Bump and Thump drill, created by head Coach Jim Copeland

Set up two cones in the center of a gym or grassy soccer field and then use the remaining cones to form a circle to identify the flow of traffic. Get two to four other riders to join you in the circle. Riders cannot take their hands off the bars or their feet off the pedals. If they dab (place a foot on the ground) or fall over, they are out. The object is to knock the other riders off their bike or make them put a foot down. The last person wins. What a hit this was with the kids! It was such a huge success that now it is the most popular drill at any of the ACA camps. The purpose is to make the rider think about their position and balance in a situation of other riders. This drill will make you think about your balance and how your position will affect you in the event of a collision.

LeMans Starts

The purpose of the LeMans Start is to teach you to control your bike in a situation when you are not on it. Start this exercise with

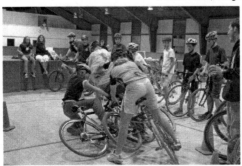

3 Cats Photo, Seliga

2004 Junior CXCamp. Competition in fierce Bump & Thump

four people at the most. Designate a finish line about 80 meters away. Line the bikes up facing the finish line, just as they would be at the start of a race. Lay the bike down on its non-drive (left) side. Designate a different start line for the riders to run from.

Run to your bike,

J. Patrick Bernard

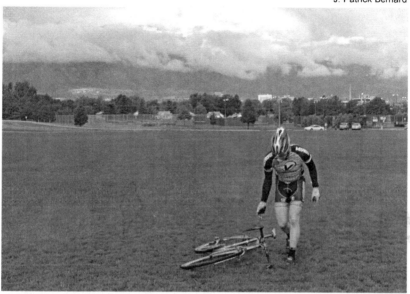

Reaching down for the grab on the handle bars.

J. Patrick Bernard

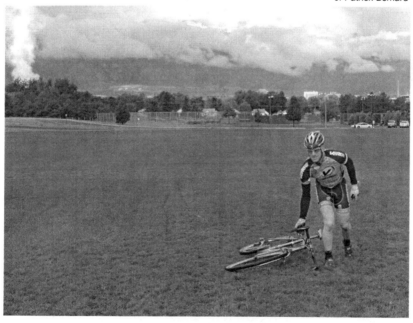

Have grabbed in the bend of the handlebars.

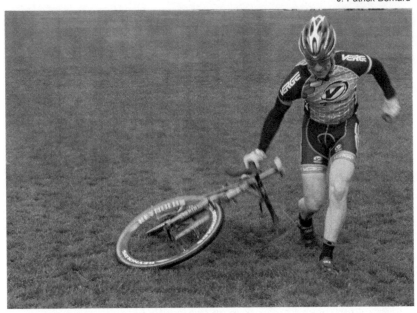

Lifting the bike up off the ground.

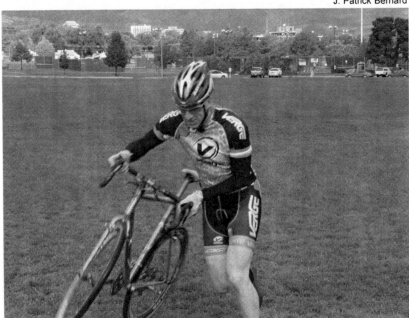

Bringing the bike up preparing for the mount.

pick it up and quickly get on. This drill emphasizes controlling the bike while running and remounting. To get the bike off the ground quickly, reach down with your hand in a scoop shape and grab the bend in the bar from the top to the curve. Bring the bike up and place it upright on the ground. Next, get on and get power to the drive train.

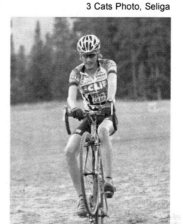

3 Cats Photo, Seliga

Wheelies

This is a good skill to practice to master your ability to control the bike. Be sure to do this on a flat, level piece of grassy ground. This way, if you fall you won't get hurt. Start by getting in your easiest gear. Ride slowly in a straight line, then pull up and back on

Kappis demonstrates at CX Camp.

the bars pulling the front wheel up. At the same time, your right leg should be applying pressure on the cranks. This torque will help bring the nose of the bike up.

At first, just get the wheel off the ground. As you feel more comfortable, get the wheel up higher and higher. This takes some practice and you will have to be in just the right gear to do this.

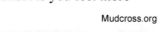

Mudcross.org

Sand Pits

In almost every cross race, I notice that the promoter loves to have a sandy section. Over in Europe they use a lot of sand in their races. Therefore, you need to practice riding the sand. Sand kills momentum, which may explain why 99% of all the racers hate the sand. So where do you find it? Many parks will have a volleyball court or a lake. Ride on the court or along the

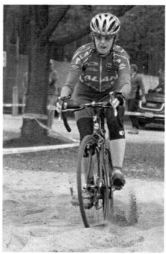

Ohio UCI, Cincinnati, Ohio

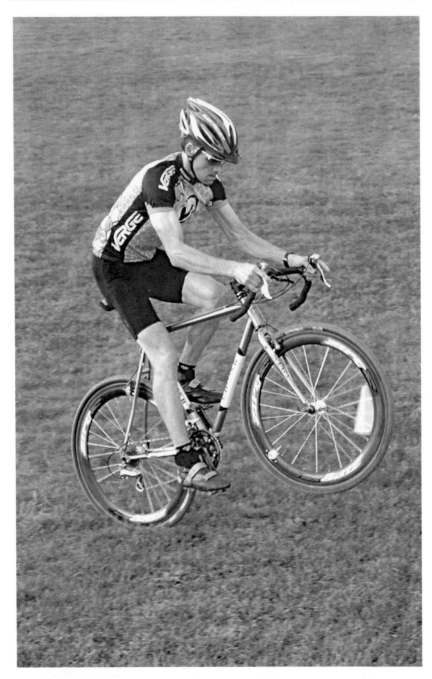

Wheelies: Great for learning balance and control.

shoreline. Start by rid-
ing a short section and
after you have mastered
that, try a longer one
until you can ride the
entire thing. A lot of
practice is necessary if
you want to be the mas-
ter of the sand and not a
victim of the sand trap.
This will build strength
and endurance. After
you have mastered rid-

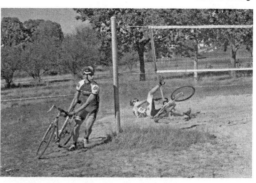

Mudcross.org

**2005 Badger Cross, Verona, Wisconsin.
Redline rider going through sand.**

ing in a straight line try turning in the sand to add to the skill. Start
with a slight change of direction and then slowly increase the size

of the turn. If
someone falls in
front of you in
the sand you will
be able to miss
them with out
having to dis-
mount or hitting
them. Things to
remember before
going into the
sand. Be in the
right gear! If you
are in the correct
gear you can
conserve your
momentum and
keep the pedals
turning. If you
don't you will
bog down, lose
all of your

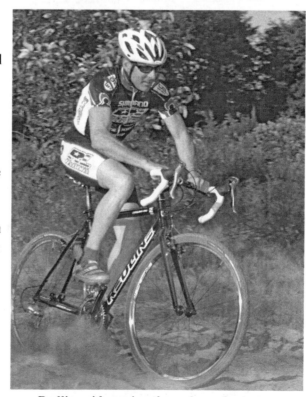

Redline rider going through sand.

momentum and stall out and fall over. Hold your line! The sand will want to make your wheel go in all different directions. Keep the wheel straight as possible. Put more of your weight on the rear wheel for more traction.

Bottle Pick-ups

Get some water bottles and space them out randomly on the ground. Ride by and try to pick up the water bottle without stopping or putting a foot down. This drill will help you with balance and bike handling and of course, come in handy if you need to pick up a water bottle in a hurry!

J. Patrick Bernard

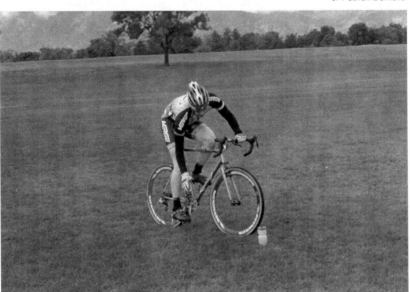

The author about to grab a bottle off the ground.

Obstacle Courses

An obstacle course gives you a chance to put all of your skills together in one final test. Combine all of the drills and put them together in a short windy course. The course should take one to three minutes to complete. It should snake back upon itself and be fun to do. Go through the course on your own a few times. When you are comfortable with the course, invite some of your friends to race it with you. Having two to four other riders on the course will help you become more comfortable riding with other riders of varying skills. Power or fitness should not be a factor, skill is the name of the game for this exercise. A LeMans Start is a creative way to begin an obstacle course.

Pit Practice

The pit is an area of the race that, while often overlooked, is an important aspect of the race. If you have not practiced going into the pits and using them, then you need to. Do you have a mechanic? If you do, practice with them and become comfortable with their style of managing this transitional area. If they happen to be experienced in a cyclocross pit, let them guide you on what will happen and how they will respond to your needs as they arise.

If you are alone and self-supported then using the pits is something that you need to practice. At one point or another, you will need to use the pit. If you have an extra bike make sure that it is set up as close to as possible to your "A" bike. The drill is to set up a mock pit and you will need to have your second bike in the pit. The bike should be facing the direction in which you are moving. Come into the pit hot and if you have a mechanic, you need to hand your old bike to them and then grab your new bike and jet off back into the race. Do this several times until it is second nature. The mechanic should catch your old bike. Have your other bike on a stand that you can just grab and go. If you don't have a mechanic, have a team mate stand in and help. Most riders can catch a bike and clean it or even change a tire or a wheel.

If you don't have a second bike and you need a wheel change, come into the pit hot and get a wheel change by you or your mechanic. First, do the front and then do the rear.

I know that this is a big pain to practice BUT doing this will ensure a couple of things. 1. When this does happen you will know exactly what to do. 2. You won't panic and make a mistake in the pit. Mistakes in the pit are time lost in the race.

You're Manning the Pit

So what do you need to do on race day? You need to know when your rider or rider's race is. Then you need to know when they need to warm up. From this you will know when you need to be there. Lets say your buddy races at 1 P.M. He or she will need to stage about 15 minutes before their race. And they will need to warm up for 30 minutes or so. This means that they need to stage at 12:45 and warm up from 12 noon. At this time. they will also need to be taking on liquids as well. They may like to warm up on the trainer or not. That's a personal choice. I would recommend a trainer and having it set up right by the starting grid. This way if it is cold your rider can stay warm till just before they start. So to the Pit! Now if the promoter is smart they will make a 2-way pit. This means that the pit will be situated in the middle of the course and the rider will pass it 2 times in the course of 1 lap. This means that they only need one pit. What you take into the pit will depend heavily on the weather. The worse the conditions the more you will have to bring with you. You will need either a spare bike or extra wheels. Maybe even both. Is it muddy? If it is or if its raining you will more than likely need a bucket and a brush with a wet lube and some tools. A 3-5 gallon bucket with some water and a long handle stiff brush will serve you well when you have to clean a bike. You will have to do this quickly as you may only have ½ a lap to get the bike ready for a exchange. A stick is also a good item to have if you have a hard time getting to some mud stuck somewhere on a brake or a derailleur. I hate it when the mud is flying and then it is drying on the bike and becomes this peanut butter / play dough that won't let go of your bike. That kind of mud seems to find its way into the smallest and most critical parts of a cyclocross bike. It will get in your chain and your pulleys on your derailleur or worse all over your brakes and start rubbing on your rims. So a nice 6" stick is a really useful tool in getting rid of that crap. Other tools that you will need are allen wrenches. This can happen even to the best of riders. Bolts come loose and stings can slip. Your handle bars can slip down or your seat post can slip down as well and when that happens that is bad news and can ruin a race for someone. I watched Ryan Trebone suffer through a series of handlebar and seat post slips in one race. I watch him pit a total of 6 times! This had a devastating effect on him and if the mechanicals had not happened he would have won the race no problem. Ryan was actually on fire that day and those mechanical problems just took the fire from his engine room.

Clothing! This is important as well as you might get dirty. Actually, I would go in expecting to get dirty. If it is raining, people normally wear rubber boots and rain coats with rain pants. You don't have the luxury of taking your time cleaning the bike. It needs to be done quickly and purposefully with out wasting time or energy. Let me put this in perspective. If it takes your buddy 7-8 minutes to do a lap, you will see them every 3-4 minutes. They can use the pit as often as they like. So they could be getting a bike change 2 times a lap if the conditions are really bad. More than likely they might take a bike every few laps if the conditions warrant it. They may come in to take a bike because they flatted a tire. Then you need to either change the wheel or give them a new bike. Quicker and easier to just give them a new bike.

Ok so now you did your duty in the pit for your buddy! Great job! So what do you do now? Well take them a jacket and a water bottle and give them a pat on the back and tell them to go and cool down. Then you need to grab the bike from the pit and anything else that you took into the pit. So let's say it was a dry day and you had no mechanicals. Then your job is pretty much done. BUT if it was wet and you had bike exchanges. you will need to clean the bike and lube the chain before you put it away Make sure you don't leave wheels or anything else in the pit. If you really want to score points have some dry clothing and some food for your buddy at the car when they get back from cooling down. A big towel and dry clothing will mean a lot to them. Food is even better! If its cold and wet something warm to drink is a lifesaver.

No Help Pit

Ok so you don't have any one helping you in the pits. So how do you do this? Well in the big races they have a area for you to lean your bike or to set your bike up. So that's easy to take care of. Just remember where you left your bike. Local races won't have all of the fancy racks for you to use. They will more than likely have a area taped off as the pit. A lot of people will be putting their wheels in, etc. I would suggest that you do get a bike stand/rack to take with you. This way your bike is not laying down on the ground for some one to step on or to run over. The rack to have will hold your bike up and it will be easy to grab on the run. I really like the super stand bike rack for this purpose. If you only have one pit and it's a 2-way pit put your bike in the middle of the pit facing perpendicular to the course. If you have it facing one direction and you need to pit and you come in from the other direction, your spare bike is facing you! Not good. If you put it facing perpendicular to the direction of the course. the bike is in a neutral position and you can grab it from either direction. I would also practice a exchange without any help. Go to a park and take both of your bikes with you and practice coming in and getting a bike.

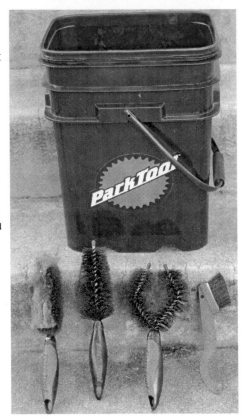

Pit bucket.

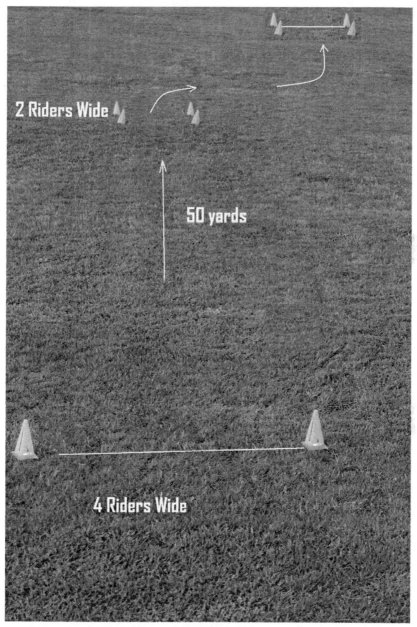

2 Riders Wide

50 yards

4 Riders Wide

Hole shot with barrier skill drill: Notice how hole shot is smaller than the start.

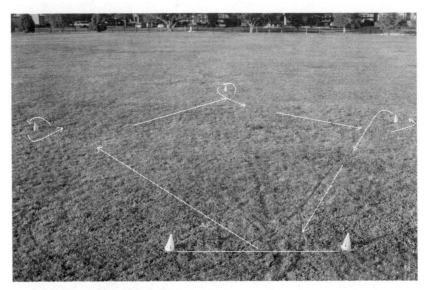

Barrel racing skill drill.

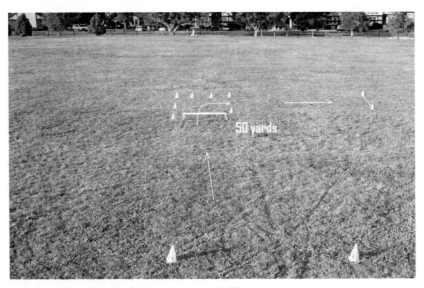

Barrier with 90 degreee corner drill.

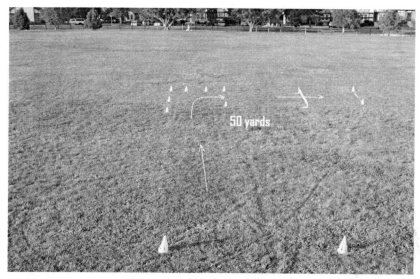

90 degree corner with barrier after.

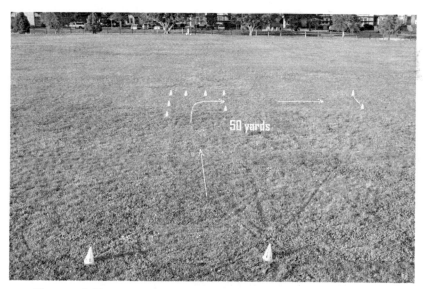

Corner drill.

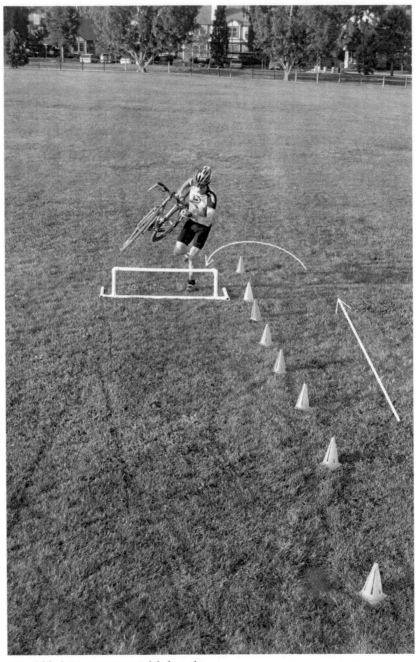

180 degree corner with barrier.

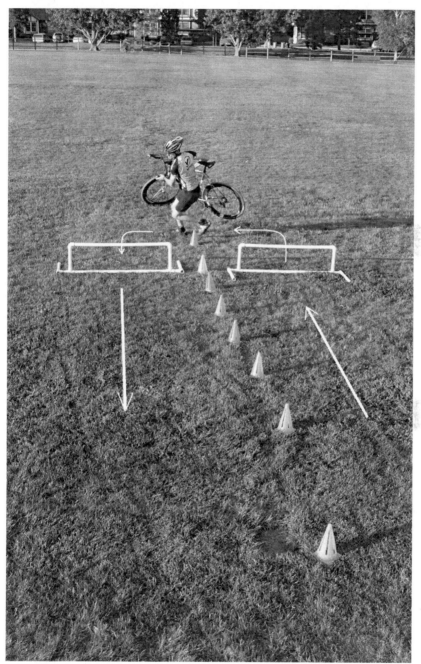

180 degree corner with barrier and after the corner.

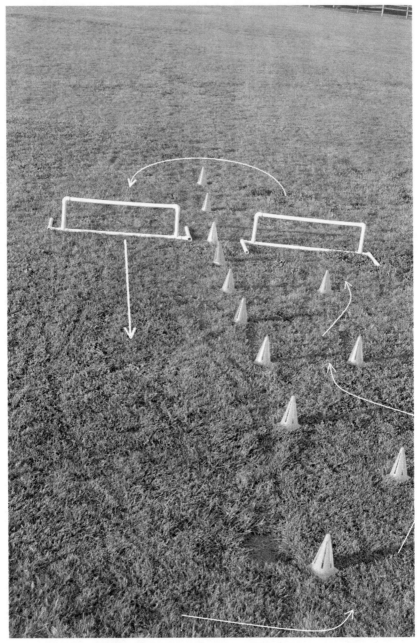

**180 degree corner with a weave drill before the
barrier/corner/barrier.**

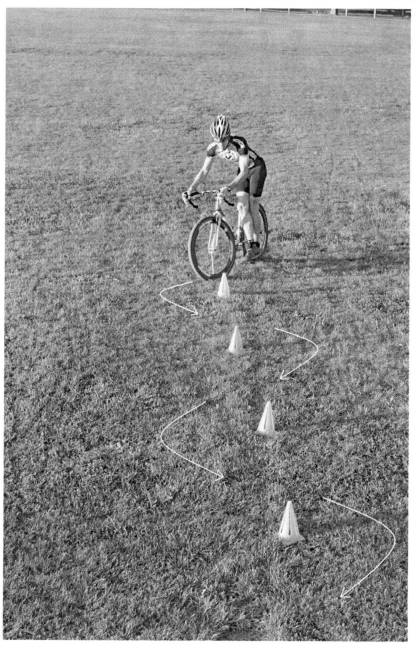

Scissor weave drill.

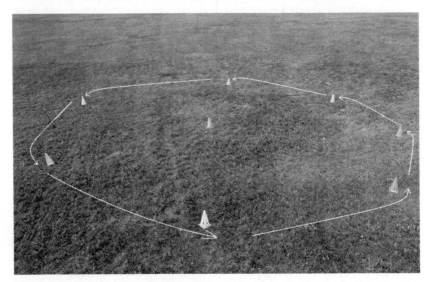

Small circle speed/corner drill.

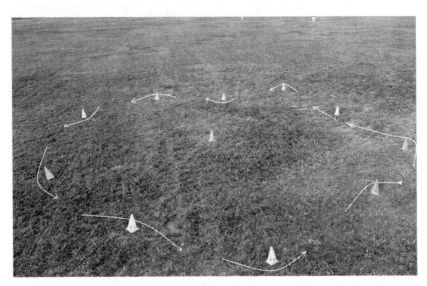

Circle speed weave/corner drill.

Making Practice Barriers

Practice barriers are very easy to make and you can even use scrap lumber that you have lying around. Regulation barriers are normally 40 cm tall and about six feet wide. Since you only need practice barriers, the dimensions will change. They need to be lightweight, durable, portable and only wide enough for two people to go over them. Practice barriers look like short wide hurdles that are "L" shaped. You should be able to place them anywhere and if you hit them, they should fall over. You can make them out of wood or PVC. If you go with PVC, head to the hardware store and use 1¼" pipe for that. At this size its pretty sturdy and light and cost effective. If you make the barriers with smaller PVC pipe it won't last getting hit or knocked over.

Here is what you will need

Item Needed	Quantity
2"X4"X5' board	1
2"X4"X 40cm (15 ¾") boards	4
½" X 2" wood screws	12
3" metal "L" brackets	2
White paint	About 2 quarts

J. Patrick Bernard

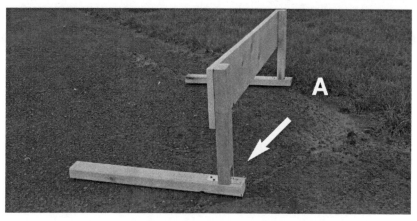

Notice the lip(A) on the barrier to keep it from falling over.

How to Assemble Your Barriers

- Step One: Base Assembly

  Take both the 40cm pieces and the 5' section

  Attach one end of the 40cm piece to the end of the 5"
  piece with screws so that the flat ends are together and
  they form a right angle.

  Repeat step to do the other side.

  Cut 1" off the 40cm legs.

- Step Two: Attach Feet to the Base

  Take the final two 40 cm pieces and measure 2" from
  the end of each one and mark a line with a pencil across
  the widest part.

  Align the back edge of the 40 cm base leg to the mark
  on the 40cm foot. This will give a 2" lip.

  Attach the 40cm foot to the bottom edge of the base
  with wood screws.

  Repeat to the other side of the base leg. Make sure that
  the feet are going the same directions. The barrier
  should look like a short hurdle.

  Now the 2" lip will be enough to keep the barrier from
  tipping over but not so much that if you hit the barrier it
  won't fall over. This barrier needs to be able to take
  some abuse.

- Step Three: Finishing Touches to Make it Last

  Attach the metal "L" brackets to the le₋ foot joint with
  wood screws. This will strengthen t'.is joint and keep it
  from breaking when the barrier i₋ dropped or knocked
  over.

  Apply a liberal amount of paint and allow it to dry.

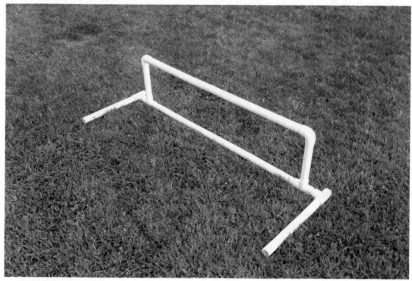

PVC barrier.

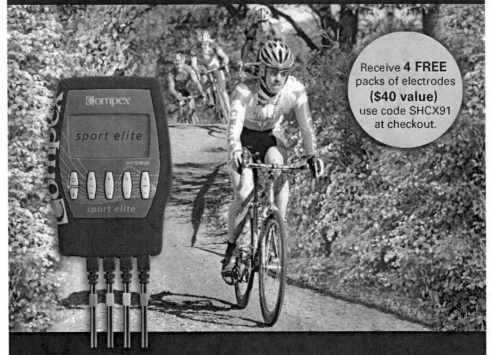

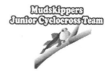

Mudskippers Junior Cyclocross Team

Beth Wrenn-Estes and Scott Mares created the The Mudskippers Junior Cyclocross Team in the fall of 2005. Erik Hultgren, the first team coach, suggested the name and the name fit the concept and so Mudskippers was born. The mission of the team was to provide younger aged kids the opportunity to enter the sport of cycling through cyclocross.

Cyclocross is a fun, laid back discipline of road cycling and includes many activities kids will love to do - jumping over barriers with a bike over your shoulder, riding in the woods or over a flat field maneuvering over obstacles and just having a good time. The discipline introduces kids to general bicycle riding skills - balance, nutrition, sportsmanship, and bicycle maintenance.

The number of juniors participating in cyclocross in Colorado had diminished and the team was a way to encourage more kids to

Margaret Fogg

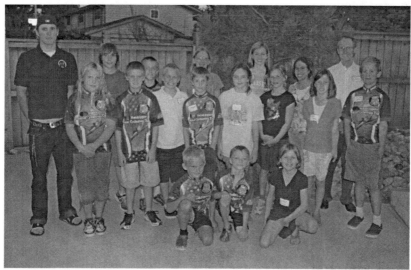

2007 Mudskipper Team Shot with Asst. Head Coach Danny Summerhill and Head Coach Dick Elliot.

participate in a non-threatening way. Beth and Scott had talked about forming a team that would be unique in composition. After speaking with several junior parents after a cyclocross camp and seeing that there was support for the idea the creation of the team moved forward quickly. One of the unique features of the team was the idea to have 10-12 year old licensed juniors but also create activities for non-licensed 8-9 year olds to participate on the team as well thus creating a way for siblings to be involved and move up to racing level when they were old enough. The competition will develop naturally but the idea behind Mudskippers continues to be one of learning about staying healthy, making friends and having.

The key to the team being successful is having a community of people involved in the effort. Parents and volunteer coaches are critical to the overall sustainability of the program. Finding sponsorship to help with the team costs is ideal and can help pay for clothing and other simple equipment needs. Approaching cycling clothing companies to support your efforts and a bike shop to help with tune-ups and parts is a simple way to make the team look professional and create a team atmosphere.. As with any sponsorship the team needs to promote their sponsors in all of the team activities. The Mudskippers team has adequate funding and provides clothing and some equipment to the each team member. Parents built the kid-friendly barriers for practices and take turns providing snacks for practices.

The team has had incredible coaches from the very beginning. Eric Hultgrin (5280) was the coach in 2006-2007 and the last two years the coach has been Dick Elliott (International Christian Cycling Club). Danny Summerhill served as an assistant coach for the team in 2007.

The idea to have Mudskippers be a "feeder" team to get kids started in the sport and then have them move onto another team is working. There are more teams of juniors racing during the cyclocross season in Colorado than there were 5 years ago. Cyclocross camps in 2006, 2007 and 2008 had over 120 juniors participating in them. The program is working and the can be developed in any part of the United States.

Program Information for Mudskippers (2008-2009)

Program purpose

To introduce boys and girls ages 8-12 to cyclocross and teach fundamentals, technique and skills that will allow them to enter JNCA cyclocross races and have fun!

Vision

To provide a fun and interesting program that will allow boys and girls to move on to sponsored cyclocross teams after racing age of 13 with the skills necessary to compete in junior cyclocross races.

Program Requirements

1. Application and acceptance on team.

2. Attend opening family picnic. Review season and schedule.

3. Attend four training sessions.

4. Attend junior cyclocross camp.

5. Race six selected cyclocross races.

6. Attend awards dinner at end of season.

7. Equipment: Team provides jersey, jacket, cycling shorts and helmet. Family provides bicycle, additional clothing and personal gear.

Team coach – Dick Elliott

I have been involved with junior road and cyclocross programs for six years. I was a coach for the junior team at International Christian Cycling Club for two years with his son Xander, who is now 21. For three years Dick was an assistant coach with Black Sheep Cycling now the head coach for the junior development program at ICCC. His son, Aaron, age 11, is on this team. Dick has a Level II USA Cycling coach certification and attends numerous coaching seminars to better understand coaching, in particular, with

Margaret Fogg

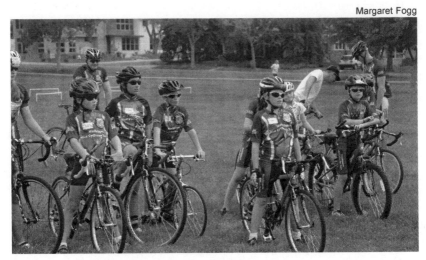

2007 Mudskippers taking instruction and practice.

junior teams. Dick is an avid road, mountain bike and cyclocross rider and frequently participates in races. He has been married to his wife Cindy for 32 years and has four children from ages 11 - 24. He is an orthodontist with a private practice in Highlands Ranch.

Dick Elliott can be reached at the following email address: dick@smilesfromtheheart.com.

Program

This is a sequential learning experience covering the following:
1. Basic rules of cyclocross.

2. Equipment: about cyclocross bikes, maintenance, adjustments, cleaning (this can be a very messy sport!), clothing.

3. Technical:

   a. Dismount, mount and carrying bicycle.
   b. Types of obstacles: hills, barriers, logs, mud pits and sand pits.
   c. Ride technique: cornering, descending, braking, bunny hopping, camber, mud, ice, snow, rocks and roots.

Margaret Fogg

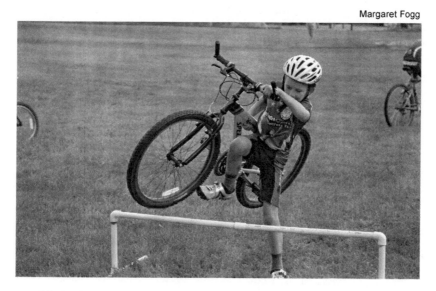

Mudskipper at practice.

4. Race

    a. Preparation.

    b. Strategies.

    c. Post race.

5. Nutrition

6. Training.

Volunteers

The program will only be as successful if parents and other caretakers volunteer. Below is a list positions needed for the team.

- Head coach – Dick Elliott

- Website/blog – Dave LaMay

- Communications coordinator (overall communications between team, parents, media) -E-mail manager (send and receive e-mails for the team) -

- ◼ Photographer (digital telephoto capability preferred)

- ◼ Newsletter Editor

- ◼ Equipment manager (transport barriers, cones, tent, etc.)

- ◼ Tent and nutrition (in charge of tent, cooler, refreshments and snacks)

- ◼ Fundraiser (solicit outside funding for the Mudskipper team)

- ◼ Parents needed to help with logistics at practices. If you ride cyclocross, bring your bike and gear to every practice. We will use you to help teach the kids. If not, we need help in the field resetting barriers, placing cones, encouraging the kids and being present with them.

Contact Beth Wrenn-Estes for more information on junior cyclocross team development at the following email address: bwestes@mac.com

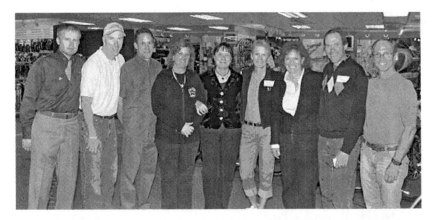

Just a few of the many people involved in junior development in Colorado. From left to right Ryan Reel (Blacksheep Cycling), Scott Mares, Jim Copeland, Karen Kincaid-Smith (Blacksheep), Beth Wrenn-Estes, Fran Summerhill, Jane Shapiro, Paul Braun (FrontRangers), Dick Elliott (Mudskippers and International Christian Cycling Team). Photo – Linard Cimermanis

Mental Training

"If you believe, you will achieve. If you doubt, you will go without."

In this section, we will discuss the different mental aspects of preparing for cyclocross competition.

Many people overlook mental training and many times we do our own mental training without even realizing it. Mental training is just one more tool in your preparation for competition.

So, what is mental training? Mental training is the training of the mind that mentally prepares you to properly deal with competition and the ever-changing situations that arise in this dynamic environment.

Mental training is not a magic pill. It will not make up for lack of physical fitness. It is not just for elite athletes and it will not fix everything right away.

Visualization

Visualizing is very important in racing. After you have walked or ridden the course and while you are warming up on a trainer, you should be riding/racing the course in your head.

Drawing a map of the course and making specific notations about specific features in each section of the course will give you a good framework upon which to build your visual training workout. For example, as you make your map, you may note the run ups, sand pits, and rock gardens. You may also make notes as to where you should watch out certain rough portions for what to avoid. However you choose to make notations about the course, the most important thing you should do with that information is formulate how and what you should be doing on that portion of the course. This may be something like "five meters before this hill, drop to 34 chain ring," or "shift down into the 26 for the climb." You may want to formulate your attack points in areas of the course that play to your strengths.

If you saw the movie "Cool Runnings," you may recall the scene where the team is in their room and they are all sitting on the floor as if they were in their bobsled. As they are sitting there, the captain is calling out the turn number and the team is reacting as they would during that turn. You may also remember the driver had photos of the racecourse that helped him remember every detail of the course. Not a bad idea, to say the least.

Another form of visualizing is actually picturing yourself racing, watching yourself lin your mind and flawlessly executing every turn, every acceleration, every barrier or remount. This will teach your body to follow your mind and is the key ingredient in the visual aspect of your mental training.

You need to also visualize how you will overcome problems that could arise in a race. Think of visualization as a rehearsal for avoiding mishaps or a mistakes during the race. Mentally going over it and seeing yourself, solving these problems will allow you to stay focused if (and when) the situation arises in the race. This kind of mental preparation will make you be seamless in these situations. Remember, mishaps and mistakes are merely a footnote, and not the entire story of your race.

To highlight the importance of mental training, I want to share this story with you. In 2006, the U.S. Grand Prix visited Boulder, Colorado. Over 3000 people attended the events. The second day was just amazing - Ryan Treborn (KONA) had easily won the race the day before. Today would prove to be even more exciting with the drama that was about to unfold.

Ryan was attacking on the hills and could pull away at will. He had power to spare. However, midway through the race, Ryan's bike developed a mechanical problem. He had to go into the pit and get a new bike. Ryan caught right back up with his breakaway companions. Unfortunately, this happened three more times in the race. This was frustrating for Ryan and he lost his desire to win. He gave up and just started riding. For several laps, the crowd watched as he merely plodded along. They soon began yelling at him to get back in the race. Finally, his mind kicked in and he went back to work. He finished that race in fourth place, but he was only 100m behind the top three. If Ryan had kept up with his mental game, he probably would have been able to bridge up to the front and win the race.

Affirmations

As cheesy as Stuart Smalley from Saturday Night Live sounded, there is some merit to re-affirming to yourself that you can do this.

Being confident is critical because it allows you to focus on the job at hand. You don't need doubt creeping into your head in the middle of a race or at the start of one. Remember, the mind can really only effectively focus on one thing. If you are filling your head with doubt, there is no room for you to visualize overcoming obstacles and finishing the race in record time.

Make up little sayings that are meaningful to you. "I can do it," "Push harder," "A little better each lap," "Everyone is hurting." These are just a few examples of what you can say to keep yourself confident and focused.

Mental Repetition and Focus

Two areas of mental repetition and focus are affirmations and visualizations. What I mean about this part is saying an affirmation or going over a movement over and over again in your head to keep it on the front of your thinking. Something like "don't go out too hard." Another one might be "stay in the top 10 to 15." You can make up your own saying that is specific to you to keep you focused and reaffirm your training and beliefs. This will help keep you calm and focused during the race. When you successfully execute a movement your confidence will grow and you will feel increasingly comfortable about the race.

Course Reconnaissance

Course reconnaissance starts with walking the course before the race and drawing it out on a piece of paper. Leave room on the page to make notes. The notes should be about which line to follow, where to ride on the course, where to get off and run, where to attack, where to recover, where to apply power etc. Then visualize the map you have created in your mind and picture the lines you will take. You can do this visualization technique while you are warming up on the trainer. After you ride the course in your head a few times on the trainer, you will be very comfortable when you're actually racing it. Also by pre-riding the course in your mind, you will not make as many mistakes. In this exercise, you should find the rhythm of the course and be able to settle into it very quickly after you start racing.

Subliminal Training

A company called Ultimate Sports Psychology has a special CD entitled "Ultimate Cyclist" that allows you to train your brain while you're sleeping. In addition to helping you get to sleep faster, you will find yourself waking up feeling better and more focused on everyday tasks. Subliminal training allows you to make the most of your time by using positive affirmations, guided imagery and progressive relaxation techniques into a CD that you can listen to while you sleep. You will find on their web site (http://www.ultimatesportspsychology.com/) that many well-known cyclists are using it in their program and are enjoying it.

Cyclocross Videos

Watching a cyclocross DVD is a great way to prepare yourself for race day. Watching cyclocross races on DVDs will not only motivate you to race, it will also help you recognize good racing tactics and techniques.

The tactics and techniques that are applied by professional cyclists tend to be more obvious when you are looking for a specific movement or technique. The pros can ride stuff that most people cannot. How did they get through those barriers so fast? How did they ride that sandy beach section? You can see how they rode through sand and then go try it. Watching these techniques and tactics and storing them in your "bank of race knowledge" will help you become a more well-rounded and efficient racer.

Ask yourself why they did certain things at different points in the race. Watch the race unfold and learn from it. Best of all you can replay something if you miss it. You can ask yourself some fundamental questions. When did they attack? When did they

Mudcross.org

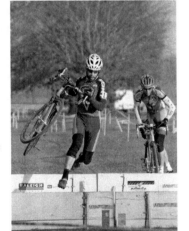

2007 Jingle Cross. A rider blazes through the barriers.

ride or run? Look at what kind of gears they are using. Watch them dismount in a barrier section. Look at how smooth they are and how they get back on. The advantage of watching the video versus watching it live (which isn't a bad idea either) is that you can play it in slow motion and replay as often as you like.

Music

Music is a great medium to utilize as part of in your mental preparation. It's best if you use music with the other parts of your routine, like your warm up and visualization time.

Goal Setting

Keeping Your Eye on the Prize

You have heard that setting goals is necessary for success. You have probably also heard that writing them down makes you 75% more likely to achieve them. You and your coach should go over your annual goals and adjust your training to align with what you want to achieve.

Goal setting is writing down specific measurable objectives that you would like to accomplish in an annual training cycle (season). There are generally four types of goals. The types are outcome short and long term, performance short and long term goals. Outcome Goals and Performance Goals: Jjust think of them as "Big Picture" Goals.. Within these goals are the short-term goals that you will need to reach those big picture goals. When you set goals you have a purpose and a place to go in your training plan. Goal setting will put you in control of your season's destination.

A good systematic goal-setting plan can:

- Improve performance

- Improve the quality of your work outs

- Help you define expectations of each work outs and direct your energy on activities that help you in competition

- Make workouts more interesting

- Motivate you to push yourself and not give up

- Increase your sense of accomplishment

Outcome Goals are goals that have a specific outcome, such as winning six races. In essence, it is the result you are training to achieve.

Performance Goals are very specific behaviors or activities that will bring you closer to achieving your Outcome Goal. Think of these as a series of performance benchmarks that will get you closer to your Outcome Goal.

Long Term Goals are goals that are set usually at the end of the season or midseason. They tend to be the final or ultimate goal of the season. They can be Performance or Outcome goals.

Short Term Goals are goals that are set to be accomplished in a short time period. They can be a weekly or a monthly goal. However, if the goal is going to take more than a month to achieve, it is not considered a Short Term Goal. Short-term goals can be either Performance or Outcome Goals.

The trick is to set Performance Goals that are in your control. Don't set goals that are out of your control. Winning a race is a goal with so many factors out of your control you cant count them. Finishing a race with specific time parameters is with in your control. This is why performance goals are better than outcome goals.

The bottom line is that you need to set a realistic measurable season goal. Follow this by setting a few midseason performance goals. These midseason goals are like base camps for climbers that ascend Mount Everest. Trying to climb the entire mountain all at once is impossible! As you reach each goal, the next one doesn't seem as daunting or unattainable.

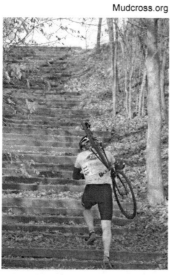
Mudcross.org

Finally, write your goals down! Review them regularly and make changes accordingly. If you see you are way ahead of a midseason goal, adjust your end of season goal so that you are still pushing yourself. Remember: Keep your eye on the prize!

A nice long run up stairs.

Intervals (Fartlek Training)

Everyone trains using intervals, right? So, how are Cyclocross intervals different? Cycling is generally classified as a non-weight bearing aerobic exercise. In Cyclocross, getting off and running with your bike, turns this into a weight bearing sport plus your bike exercise..

The transition from the efficient bike ride to the inefficient run puts an overload on your system, one that you must train your body to become accustomed to. This sudden overload to the system can take you from "on the border" to "over the edge" physically and mentally if you do not implement steps in your training to prepare for it.

The principle of specificity is part of the FITT principle of training. FITT stands for Frequency, Intensity, Time and Type. The FITT principle can be applied to any sport, but for our purposes, we will focus on how this principle applies to cyclocross intervals.

A cyclocross interval should have three sections to it: – before the run, during the run and after the run. These intervals will address demands that are unique in a cyclocross race. These intervals will be mostly ride/run/ride intervals.

LT Intervals

Lactate Threshold (LT) is the most simple and basic of the intervals. Once you have been tested, your coach can determine your LT. LT intervals can be done in a variety of ways. The only component that changes is the time of each interval. Normal LT intervals will last anywhere from 10 to 20 minutes in length. These can be done on either a steady climb or an open road. Your coach will tell you the frequency, intensity, and the duration of these intervals.

VO2 Intervals

VO_2 max (also called maximal oxygen consumption, maximal oxygen uptake or aerobic capacity) is the maximum capacity of an individual's body to transport and utilize oxygen during incremental exercise, which reflects the physical fitness of the individual.

The name is derived from V - volume per time, O_2 - oxygen, max

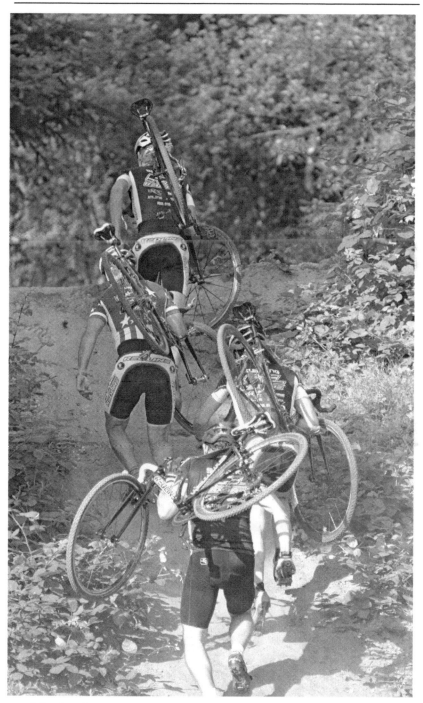

The Redline train takes a run up.

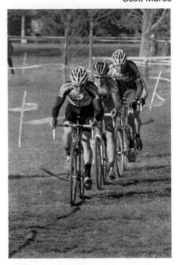
Scott Mares

2007 Boulder Super Cup.

- maximum. This is the hardest of the single types of intervals and requires plenty of base work and preparation. Your coach will determine your VO_2 range by either wattage or heart rate. VO_2 efforts will allow the rider to increase the maximum amount of volume uptake of Oxygen. Too much training at this level will negatively affect your performance.

LT and VO_2 Intervals

LT and VO_2 intervals will probably be the most useful in your race preparation. In this interval you will start out with an LT effort for short period of about five minutes then switch to a VO_2 max effort for one minute, then switch back to another LT effort for another five. This combination is repeated. This is to simulate race situation of racing and then attacking and then back to race pace.

Race Starts

Simulating the start of a cyclocross race is very important because your placement in the first kilometer will determine a lot of your strategy and tactics for the remainder of the race. You must be aggressive, but not overextend yourself. The way you start the race will determine your strategy. You do not want to overextend yourself at the start of a race. Otherwise, it could take you the entire length of the race to try to recover from a poorly executed start.

Find a place where you can set up a course for a start simulation. These intervals should consist of a long straight away followed by several sections of twisty turns. Off-camber, single track, and steep descents should be included in your practice course as well.

A race start interval should be started after a good warm up. Find your start and come to a complete stop. Start just as you would start in a race. If you have a couple of your friends to participate with you, it will make this interval more realistic and force you to tweak your start strategy accordingly. This interval is only one minute in length.

Strength Endurance

This interval is easiest to do on the trainer. Set the resistance very high so that you are riding at about 50 RPMs. Start out at five minutes on and five minutes off. Increase your interval time as you increase in strength and endurance.

Race Sections

This is another way to do your intervals for the cross season. Set up your own cross course, complete with the usual running sections. The interval consists of doing one minute of LT effort, 30 seconds of running and one minute of LT effort. Recover for one to two minutes after each interval.

Sand Pit Intervals

Once you have found a sandy section or a volleyball court to practice riding in the sand, you can do intervals in it. These will be power intervals.

Scott Mares

2007 Boulder Cup. Frank Hibbits lays down the power in the sand.

Ride-Sand Run-Ride

This interval is simply riding at race pace for one minute, running in the sand for 30 seconds, and then riding for another minute. Follow this up with a recovery. This will help your running power and your power after a run.

Riding in the Sand

Start the interval with riding in regular 'cross-terrain for one minute at race pace. Continue riding into a sand pit another minute, and then continue back to regular terrain. This interval is ridden throughout its entirety. Do not dismount. This will build power and bike handling skills. This will also give you confidence in races where you can ride the sand pit, which is faster than running it.

Margaret Fogg

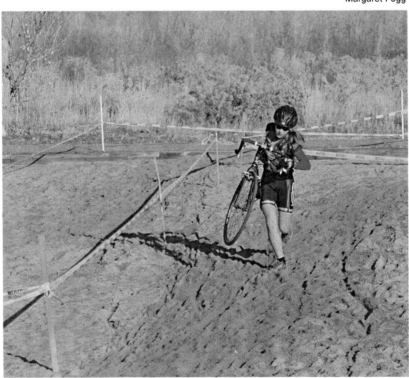

Mud Skipper Taylor Fogg running through sand at a Boulder race.

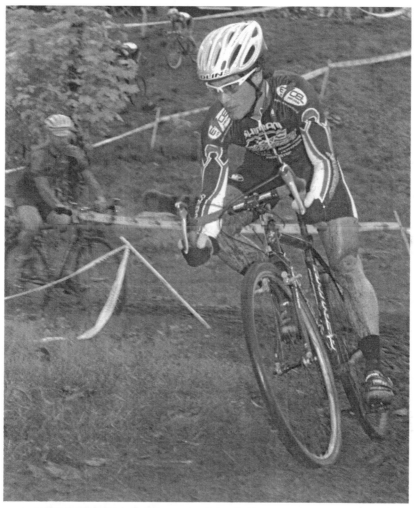

Redline rider Dave Richter in full flight in the great Northwest.

Ride-Barrier/Hill-Ride

Taking the section of a racecourse and use it as your interval. You can do this on a flat section or you can do this on a hill. You can change the interval to run the entire hill or run some of it, then ride the rest in the appropriate gear to accelerate back up to race speed.

Start this exercise on the flats. After you have done a few sets on the flats, do the interval with the hills next. However, it will do you no good if you attempt a hill that exceeds your current level of fitness. Too much OR too many intervals and your fitness will start to go backwards.

Ride-Barrier/Hill-Ride (Over Geared)

This interval simulates situations where you have ridden up to a barrier section, gotten off, and remounted in a gear that is too big. Simulating this situation in interval format will help with your power after running. You can vary this type of interval by doing it on a flat section or on a hill. Vary it even more by running part of the hill then riding the rest of it over geared.

I would like to reinforce that the intervals must comply with the "FITT" principle (Frequency, Intensity, Time and Type). I did not put in how long (time) or how often (frequency) the intervals should be because this is very individualistic and should be prescribed by a certified coach. Intervals are a great way to train but be careful not to do too much too often where you become over trained and slow.

Tactics

The tactics of a cyclocross race are just as different as in road, track and mountain bike racing. However, it's the same formula as to how you figure out what you need to do.

Scouting the Course

Scouting the course is very important in your race preparation. Before the race, ride the course and see how it is laid out. Watch how other people are riding the different sections. What line are they taking in each section? Try those lines and then ask yourself, "Is that the best line?" If not, try other lines. The more you scout, the better you're going to be in a race. This will also give you an opportunity to determine what tire pressure you need to run. Your tire pressure is very important in a race. You want to have the optional amount of traction to go as fast as you can. This is discussed in later chapters.

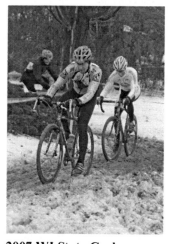

2007 WI State Cyclocross, Hales Corner, Wisconsin. Mother nature can make things interesting by giving you snow and ice to race in.

The timing of your scouting session is very important as well. The course will change throughout the day. Especially if it becomes wet or there is a big temperature change.

On December 3, 2006, the Red Rocks Cyclocross Race in Morrison, Colorado, got 6" of snow. In the morning, the course was powder snow and ice. By the time the senior open race started, the course had changed to soupy mud with no ice in sight. The temperature went from 25° to 38° F over the course of the day.

This is a great example of what can happen over time to a race course. The course can change even more with steady rain. If the course is under constant rain, you can bet there will be a lot of erosion. If you scout the course too early it may look completely different by the time you actually race it. There may be new ruts and the paths may be different. In addition, you may need to change your tire pressure. The course could be more slick than when you first rode it. You may even need to change out your original choice of tires.

Going From the Front

If you have a great start and you don't fade, then going from the front is a good bet. Going from the front is advantageous because you are less likely to be caught behind all the mistakes of the riders in front of you, bottlenecks, and traffic.

If there are 60 racers in the race and you don't want to be in the bottleneck at the start of the race, go from the front. The strongest rider can lose a race if they are caught up in a bottleneck and are stuck in traffic. Here's the other side to this tactic - if you go too hard, you can blow up and end up spending a few laps just trying to recover from the way you pushed yourself at the start.

Attack the Run Ups

Are you a good runner? It's very hard to go from a non-weight bearing aerobic situation to a weight bearing plus a bike then back again. Once again, if you overextend yourself on a run-up, you are not going to be moving forward. However, if you are an efficient runner and can force the other riders to overextend to keep up with you, then run-ups are a great opportunity for you to increase your advantage. If you are with someone, look to see if he/she is a good runner. If your competition is struggling on the run-ups and recovery, this is a good indication that you should attack them on the run-ups.

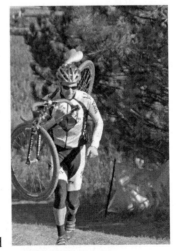

Mudcross.org

2007 Kletsch Park Cyclocross, Milwaukee. By running early and often in the season, you can make huge gains in a race.

Attack the Barriers

Are you good on the barriers? Can you take them faster than anyone else?

If you can, push the pace through the barriers.Make your competitors make a mistake and hit a barrier.. The faster you go, the less of a margin for error you have. This means you have to bring your "A" game into your timing on your techniques. If you do, the rewards can be big. Smart cyclocross riders know their limits and will not be pressured by other riders to overextend themselves. Instead, they will look to gain ground in a different section.

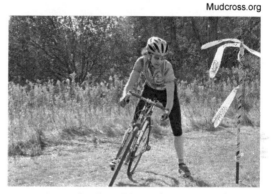

Mudcross.org

2006 Lapham Park Cyclocross, Delafield, Wisconsin.

Attack the Technical Section

Do you have great turning skills? Pushing the pace through these sections is a great way to play into your strengths. These sections may make a less experienced rider bobble, crash or overshoot a corner. If you have better tires or gears, the course and weather may be your advantage.

Attack the Sand Pit

Every promoter likes to put a sand pit in his or her race. Think of this section as a sand trap for your competition. Sand pits have a way of zapping the energy out of even the fittest legs. People sink in it and it takes away forward momentum. You get less traction and now you have to decide: Do I run or ride this section? If you get a straight shot, pick some 34 tires and ride it, if the approach is at a 90-degree corner, you may have to run it.

The Europeans have a lot of sand in their races. If you look online, you will see them riding in it all the time. They have a lot of power and know how to ride the sand. Having 34's doesn't seem to hurt either.

Stalking

Stalking is a tactic to use when you are strong enough to let other people go out and overextend themselves, allowing them to make mistakes. In this tactic, you follow wheels and sit in the second or third position. You chase the attacks but wait to counter in the latter parts of the race. To do this, you must be the strongest and very patient.

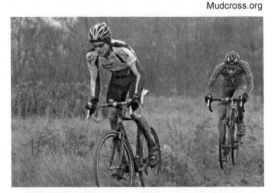

Mudcross.org

2006Trash Dash Cyclocross, Whiterwater, Wisconsin. Soft gravel will suck the energy from you. Having good endurance is essential in cyclocross.

When you decide to jump depends on how long you can sustain an attacking effort. Knowing whether you can go from the gun or just stalk the competition for half of the race will determine your strategy if you plan to use this tactic. To use this tactic, it is imperative that you evaluate your competition and see where everyone is at in regards to his or her abilities and level of fitness.

Ride or Run

Now for the $100,000 question: Is it faster to run or ride? Try riding and then running it. The answer just might surprise you. The most important thing to consider is how much of a toll is running or riding that section going to take on you physically. If it is faster to ride, but you find yourself struggling to recover, it may be better to run that portion.

Energy expenditure is like a book of matches. When you begin the race, you only have a set number to burn. Riding up a hill may cost you two matches, but you may spend more time recovering than if you ran up. This is why doing a thorough course reconnaissance is so critical to your success in every race.

Equipment Selection

Equipment can often be the difference between winning and

finishing. The most crucial decision you will make is tire selection. The right rubber and pressure can make all the difference. Of course, tire selection is highly dependent on the course conditions and layout. Is it steep with hard corners or all grass with good grip? So...what about snow and ice? Do you have snow tires or ice tires? You won't use them very often. However, I recommend you get one set of snow/ice tires. You will only use them once or twice a year so they will last you a lifetime of cyclocross and winter riding. When you do use them, they are very useful. The traction that they provide can be the difference between staying up and spitting mud and ice from your mouth. I have a couple of pairs of these tires. The traction that they provide is amazing. The trade off is that they are heavy.

Your Competition

Your competition will influence much of what you do both before and during your race, probably more so than any other factor. One of the most important things you can do for yourself is pay attention to your competition and what they are doing and when/where they struggle. Now this may not be obvious at first, but the signs may be very subtle and you will have to know what to look for. Be watchful of any place that your competition is not fluid and just as importantly, any place that you have a clear advantage in terms of strength or skill.

Inge Wortman

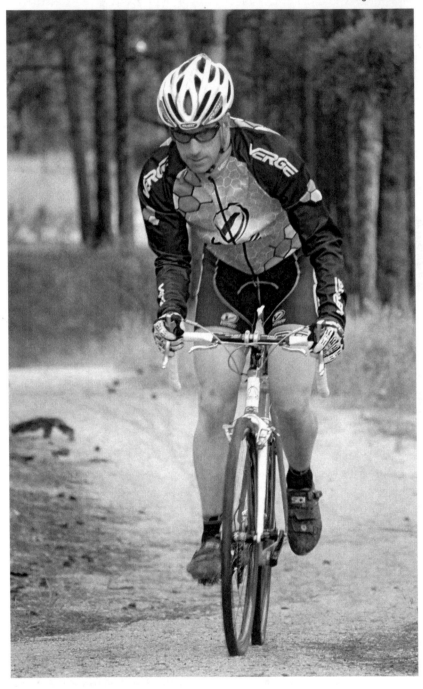

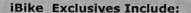
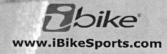

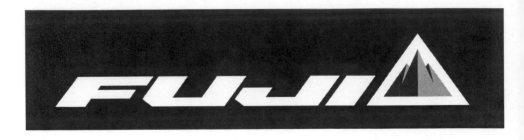

CROSS PRO

A-6 aluminum frame
FC-770 carbon fork
Shimano Ultegra SL components
Mavic Aksium Race wheelset

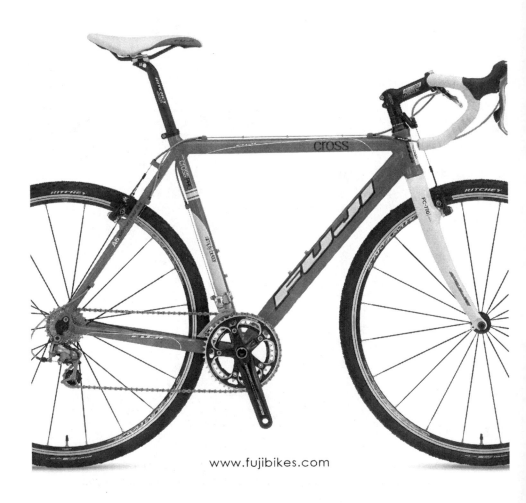

www.fujibikes.com

Warm Up

Warming up is just as important as studying the course and selecting the right equipment. Without a good warm up, it will take you the first half of the race to get into the groove. Consequently, you will spend the first half trying not to go into the red zone.

Scott Mares

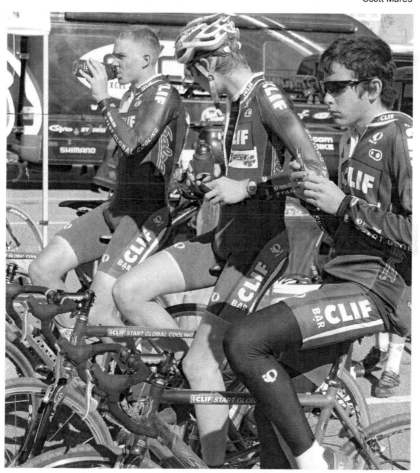

Warm up at Boulder race. Would you go to race your car and NOT put gas in your tank? NO ... So fuel up and warm up so you can be ready at the gun.

There should be a couple of parts to your warm up. The first is on the course. This means that you are warming up on the course and practicing the course at the same time. Seeing which line to take and how to take the barriers and run ups. This is also called mapping.

The second half of the warm up is just that, warming up. One of the better choices is to use a rim trainer like the Minoura rim trainer. Other trainers get resistance from tire contact, which will place undue wear on your cyclocross tires. If you don't have a rim trainer any trainer will do, however, you may want a extra wheel just for the trainer. They make tires just for trainers now and they last a long time.

Equipment

Let's take look at all of the types of gear that goes into cyclocross. This will include frames, forks, wheels, gears, cranks, tires and so forth.

The Bike

A cyclocross bike will look like a standard road bike, but have some subtle differences. The most obvious difference is that the tires are larger and have traction knobbies on them. You can also see that the bike has canti or disc brakes. Other than these two differences, a cyclocross bike looks very much like a regular road bike.

Scott Mares

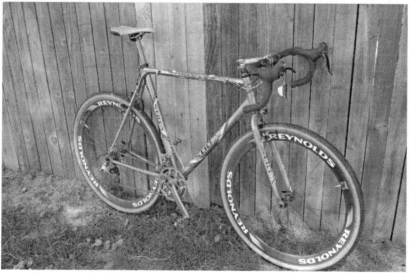

The author's bike.

Frame

The frame is the heart of the bike and if you have a cyclocross-specific frame, you will be much happier in a cyclocross race. There are different makes of cyclocross bikes all with varying component materials. Although there is much debate over which materials are best, you will find that with any material, there will *always* be a trade off. This trade-off will be in weight, price or strength. Usually you can pick two of the three. The most common materials that frames are made out of are steel, carbon fiber, aluminum and titanium.

Scott Mares

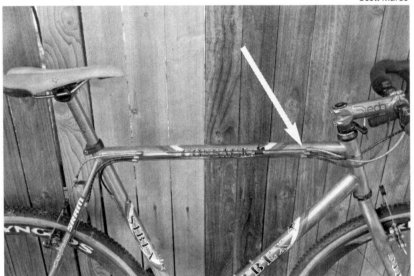

Notice the cables are routed on the top tube and on the side.

Steel is a great material. It's strong and is easy to work with. It is extremely durable. The drawback however, is its weight - it can be very heavy. However, with new emerging technologies, that is changing. Steel, like all the other materials, is evolving with new alloys and treatments. Twenty years ago, Columbus had the cutting edge with their SL tubing. Today, there are several types of steel that are lighter and stronger. Reynolds 953 and FOCO tubing are just two examples of the evolution of steel.

Carbon fiber is an impressive material. It is light, strong and you can shape it into different forms. It tends to be a bit pricier than aluminum and steel, and is more susceptible to impact and moisture.

Aluminum or Aluminum/carbon fiber is another available material. Now remember there is always a trade off with any materials. Aluminum is a great material because you can shape it and form it easily. It's cheap and light. However, the trade off is that it transmits everything to the rider. In addition, it's a one or two season material. You can paint it and it won't rust. Most bike companies manufacture aluminum frames, making them more common and less costly.

Titanium is considered the "Holy Grail" of material for Cyclocross and, in my opinion, is one of the better materials for a cyclocross frame. It's stiff but comfortable. It doesn't rust, and it's very lightweight and durable. However, there are still limitations with this material. It's hard to come by and difficult to work with and shape. It is still pricier than other materials.

Forks

There are many good cyclocross forks on the market right now. Some are made of carbon fiber, but most are steel, aluminum or even titanium. The most important thing to consider when purchasing a fork for a 'cross bike is the reputation of the brand. Not all carbon cross forks are equal. Some have aluminum steer tubes and some come have carbon ones. However, my personal favorite is full titanium - light, durable and a great ride.

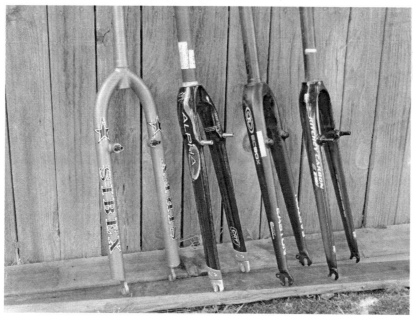

Just some examples of the great forks available in the CX market.

Handlebars

Handlebars are a component that is largely one of personal choice for the rider. However, you should consider some things like the shape of the bar and the positioning of the levers. Ideally, you should have the same size bars as you have on your road bike.

Recently, bars are being made with flattened tops. This provides a comfortable position for the hands on the top of the bars. However, if you like the extra top break levers, this can pose a problem. The shape of this type of bar does not lend itself to mounting top mount levers in a good position. The placement would require them to be very close to the stem, which is bad for handling since moving your hands inward reduces the stability and leverage you have in handling.

The materials used to manufacture handlebars are evolving just as quickly as every other bike component. They used to be made out of steel, then aluminum and now carbon fiber. Since carbon fiber has been out on the market for a while, the ones out there are well designed and very strong.

Now this is not to say that aluminum bars have not developed over the years. Currently there are several good, light aluminum handlebars on the market. Deda® makes a very light and strong aluminum handle bar. Again, the technology for making different alloys in aluminum has evolved with time giving way to better and very cost-effective components.

Wheels

The choice of wheels can have the biggest impact on a cyclocross bike's performance. The wheels not only will make the bike weigh less, but help in acceleration and aerodynamics. There are two categories of wheels: tubulars and clinchers. The true cyclocross racer will go with tubulars. They are lighter and you can run a lower tire pressure. Tubulars are a little more trouble but the ride is better. It used to be if you got a flat you had to get it repaired. Now you can get tubulars that accept the sealant by TUFO. That means that you just need to have a tube of the sealant handy to fix your tubular tire.

Currently the hottest wheel on the market is a carbon tubular of

Scott Mares

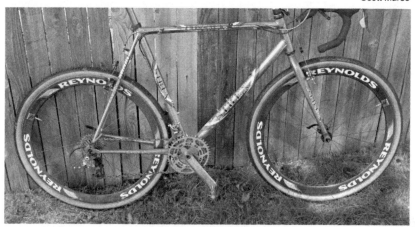

The wheels of choice. Reynolds DV46 Cross Wheelset.

the Zipp 303 variety. This wheel is in the 1200 to 1400 gram range. It's a mid deep rim that is very desirable because of the low weight and ease of acceleration. The mid deep rim is good for sand and mud. When a wheel sinks in sand, a regular rim will have sand on top of the rim and will be covered. The aero rim does not allow the sand to get on top of it and keeps the sand at bay. The rims are not only aerodynamic, but strong as well. My personal favorite in this category is the Reynolds DV46. When used with DT Swiss hubs, it is light and stronger than ZIPPs. Reynolds also offers a great replacement program. The clincher version of this would be the American classic CR420's. These wheels are very light for clinchers and are also a mid section aero wheel.

Tires

Tubular: My favorite tire is the Challenge Grifo. The 2007 version has an extra row of dots on the outer edge for increased edging. I like the Grifo because of the better cornering and the suppleness of the tire. TUFO has made a new tire called the Flexus, which seems to be a very good tire with its extra row of tread for better edging. However, this is the only tire the TUFO line has with the extra row of tread for edging. All of the Grifo tires have the extra tread on the sides. Plus, you can get the Grifo in more sizes. I believe that TUFO will listen to consumer demand and offer the

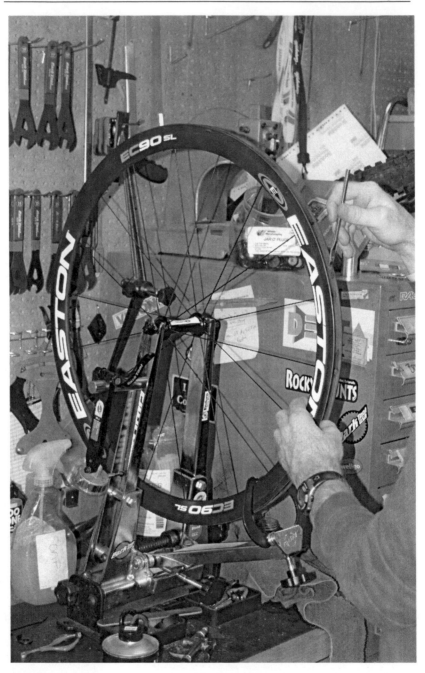

Putting the wheel on a stand is the eay way to paint the glue on a wheel.

extra tread in all of their versions of cyclocross tires that they offer. TUFO does have the largest selection of cyclocross tires

Clinchers: Again I would have to pick the Grifo, since they ride like a tubular. However, there are many clincher tires being made, like the ones Michelin makes for muddy and dry conditions.

Arctic/Winter conditions require special tires. Innova makes an ice and snow tire with a wide chevron tread pattern and small studs for icy conditions. They are heavy, but they provide a tremendous amount of traction. This pattern is deep and cleans very quickly. They provide excellent traction in the snow and especially on the ice. I was very impressed with the traction I got on an off camber decent in a race in Morrison, Colorado. They had six inches of snow the night before and I was able to descend on this off camber section at twice the speed of my competitors. People were falling and crashing all over the place because they had the wrong tires.

Size matters

The size of the tire does matter. The skinnier the tire, the lower the rolling resistance and thus the faster it is. However, the trade off is that you are sacrificing ride quality and traction in cornering

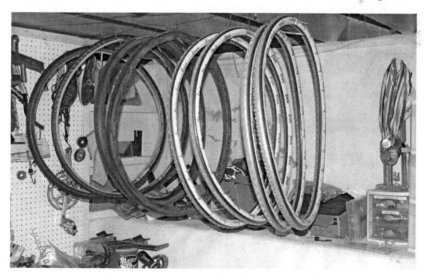

When you're gluing tires, hang them up to dry.

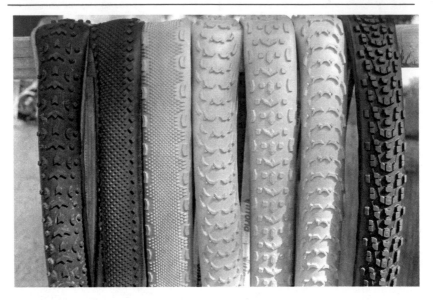

There are lots of tires with several tread patterns available now.

(edging). The larger the tire the better the edging and ride quality, which means you will sacrifice a little on speed. However, the bigger the tire, the lower the pressure you can run. Tires run from as small as 28c up to 35c. Most people race 32c and 34c. This width will give you the best in traction and rolling resistance while keeping weight down. The 35c are usually specialty tires for snow and ice.

Rubber

The harder the rubber, the faster it is. However, the harder it is, the less pliable it will be. That means that it won't conform to the ground when edging or going over rough terrain. More supple tires are usually best, but generally do not last more than one or two seasons. The higher quality tires will have different tires for different weather conditions. Usually the manufacturer will use a different color for different uses. The manufacturer may even change the tread pattern as well.

Tread Patterns

Because cyclocross is becoming more and more popular in the US, there are more and more companies making cyclocross tires. All of these companies are making tires in different tread patterns, choosing the right pattern is one of the most important choices other than the size of the tire. Most tubular tires will have a center tread pattern of arrows. The important element to look for is how far do the side knobs go and how many of them there are. After all, the side knobs provide your traction in edging.

The next consideration is how does the tire clear itself? Well you can't ask the manufacturer because they will tell you that their tread clears mud. So the next best thing to do is to take a look at what other people have and how their tires respond to the environment. There are specific mud tires with special tread for muddy conditions.

As I mentioned before, Michelin makes a set for dry (Jets) and muddy (Mud) conditions. The jets have a file-diamond tread pattern with raised side tread for edging in dry conditions. The mud tire has special tread for traction and clearing mud from the tire. The traditional arrow and dots are considered by most the best for all conditions.

Tire Pressure

Tire pressure is very subjective and there are many variables that determine correct tire pressure. So why is this so important? Two reasons: traction and ride quality. Most importantly - traction, traction and more traction. You can't win if you don't stay upright. So, what's the magic formula? There is none but the key contributing factors are the rider's weight, the type of tire they are using (rubber and tread pattern), the size of the tire (30c, 32c, 34c or 35c), the course terrain and the weather conditions. All of this will need to be considered when determining the correct tire pressure.

Traction

If you have a high tire pressure, you have low rolling resistance and a very fast tire. However, you sacrifice traction. This does not mean you will have bad traction in less than ideal conditions. You can sacrifice this in dry and 70 degree conditions. It's the terrain that influences this. So, is the grass long, short, wet, dry, or dead? Are you racing on dirt, mud, decomposed granite, concrete, asphalt, or cinder? What is the temperature? Is it 20 degrees or 70 degrees outside?

Why does a lower tire pressure give you better traction? Simple, the lower tire pressure allows the tire to conform to the terrain. This is called the footprint. The larger the footprint, the better the traction will be. Conversely, the higher the tire pressure, the less the footprint (and traction) will be.

So what do you want? You want your tire pressure low enough to give you good traction in the corners and high enough so you won't bottom out on the course.

How do you get that ideal tire pressure? Don't try to get it at the race on race day for the first time. Just like all new race equipment, try it out *before* the race. Go to your favorite cyclocross course and start with 50psi in your tires. Take a lap, then let a little air out before taking another lap. Repeat this until you feel that the bike is on the edge of being out of control. At this point, add small amounts of air to the tires until you reach the best tire pressure for that course. Once you have gone through this, you can adjust your tire pressure on race day after one or two laps.

Shifters

Over the past years, shifters were primarily either Shimano or Campy. Recently, there has been an equally impressive third choice, SRAM. Most of the bikes will have this style shifter. Of course, the old school rider can still use the bar end shifters. Again, this is choice of personal taste and comfort. Many times athletes just become comfortable with one brand and have difficulty adjusting to anything else.

Cranks

In the past, cyclocross riders had to use a standard road crank for their cyclocross bikes. That is not the case anymore. Now, a compact crank is the crank of choice This means that the BCD (Bolt Chain ring Diameter) is 110mm. A standard crank has a 130 BCD. The compact crank allows you to run the proper chain ring size for

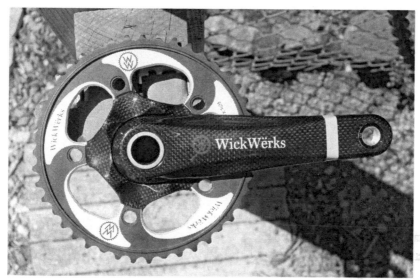

Wick Werks carbon crank.

your ability. The standard crank is limited by how small of a chain ring can be mounted on it.. Most of the component manufacturers make a 110 BCD crank, so why would you choose a 110 crank instead? Simple, if you use a compact crank, you can run a 46X36 and not be over geared. This crank will also give you the flexibility

Scott Mares

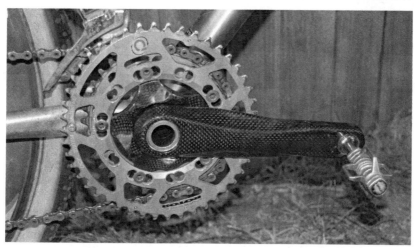

Carbon Cranks and Q-rings are more and more common. Q-rings will give you an extra 4% power in your pedal stroke.

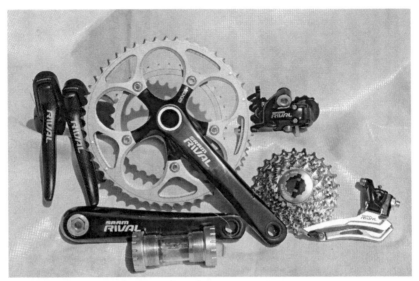

For the money the best CX group on the market.

to run a wide range of gears as apposed to a 130BCD crank. If
you're strong enough, you can run a larger ratio or a single ring
with guards.

There have been many changes in crank technology in the past
10 years. Most cranks were either steel or aluminum. Then they
were made of aluminum. Now carbon fiber has started taking up
large chunks of the market. Now, it's not uncommon to see cranks
made out of carbon fiber, even in a compact version.

Chain Rings

There are several options available on the market today. You
can choose to go with a single or double chain ring. So, what is the
best size? The answer to that question depends solely on you and
your strengths.

Going compact double is a common way to go. This combination is a 46X36 set up. This can be found on several cranks that are
available in the market. Now you have to remember that the crank
is a 110 BCD. Standard road cranks are 130 BCD, except for
Campy. The advantage is that you can run a wider range of gearing
with a 110 versus a 130 BCD crank. You can only go to a 38-tooth
small chain ring.

If you wanted, you could get your old chain rings from your road bike. If you choose to go with a single ring, you can take an old 52 and grind off all the teeth to have a chain guide - You would just need to get some MTB bolts and some spacers.

However, I have chosen to go with the Rotor Q ring set up. The Q rings are NOT Bio Pace. Several years ago, Shimano came out with Bio-pace and they did not work as advertised. Rotor, a company in Spain did the proper research and came out with a fully adjustable elliptical chain ring to give you mechanical advantage in your pedaling mechanics. The advantage is you will get about a 4% increase in power with these rings.

The other chain ring I would highly recommend is made in the USA by Wick Werks. These rings are really awesome in that they have taken shifting to the next level. A normal chain ring grabs the chain when you shift it by a pin or a very small ramp. This means it grabs the chain by a single pont. The Wick Werks rings are radically ramped. They grab a total of 3 links when you shift. What does this mean? You can shift under any load, any rpm. I was really impressed with they way they performed. As the saying goes: strength, weight, price. You can choose only 2 of the 3. Not in this case. They are lighter, stronger, and cheaper than XTR. So when

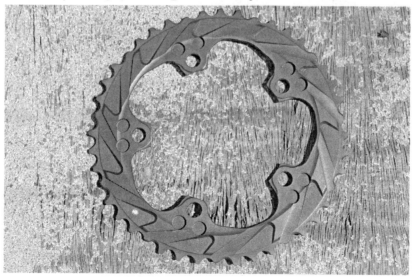

Notice the radical ramping on the rings.

you have a speed change and you need to shift right now, these are the way to go.

Bottom Bracket

This is pretty much the same choice that you would have for your road bike. FSA titanium platinum pro is a good choice if you go ISIS. Another one is the American Classic BB. This is one of the lightest ones available. If you go with an external bottom bracket, any of the major brands will do. FSA does make one with ceramic bearings in it. If you go with an external bottom bracket, you will be limiting your options if you decide to go with a compact crank. Technology is changing all of the time in cycling and all you have to do is wait a little bit. For instance, Shimano just came out with D/A compact cranks. The external bottom brackets are very easy to install and don't require adjusting at all. Just prep the threads, screw the cups on, and then install the cranks. Its really that simple.

Derailleur

A long time ago, you could choose what kind of derailleur you wanted. However, current systems require a derailleur that is the same brand as your shifters. Until recently, Campy or Shimano were the only choices. Now SRAM and some other smaller manufacturers have entered the fray. Either way, you will want to make sure that your derailleur can handle the size of the largest cog in your cassette. This will be a choice of taste and not one from a rule.

Cassette

The cassette should reflect where you race. In Colorado it's mostly vertical so it's pretty standard to run a 11X26 or a 12X26 cassette. Choose your own poison based on your region, strengths and skill level.

Brakes

There are many different brakes for cyclocross that are available on the market, and until recently, the UCI had banned the use of disc brakes. The most common brake for cyclocross is the cantilever brake. Several companies make good brakes, such as Spooky, Avid, Tetxtro, Paul and Shimano. Some offer adjustability and some have a better travel than the others. Some are lighter than others. However, remember, with equipment there is always going to be a trade off in one of three areas:weight, strength and price. Weight weenies will want the spooky and other carbon types of brakes. If your concern is weight then the spooky and frogs are the choice. If you want performance, weight and adjustability then the Tetxtros are the clear choice.

Shoes

This is a very important and personal piece of equipment. Ideally, you want a shoe that has a stiff but flexible sole. If the shoe is too stiff, it's not good for running. If it's too soft, it's not good for cycling. My favorite is the Sidi Dominator. Just like wheels, you are going to want to have a few pairs of these shoes. If possible, you should have a summer version, wet fall version and then a winter/arctic version.

The summer version should have breathable mesh that will allow your foot to breathe in warm weather riding/racing. You can't control the weather, but if you have the right clothing, it can make your race a lot more comfortable. Fall can have a wide range of weather, so your fall shoe should be full leather or synthetic leather.

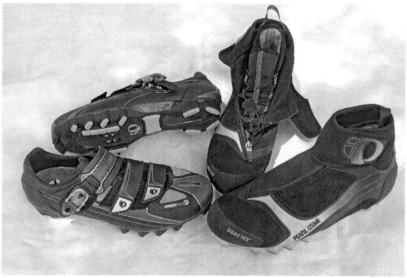

A regular set and a winter set of CX shoes is a really good idea.

This will keep your foot more comfortable in the different weather conditions. When the weather turns cool and wet this type of shoe will keep out the cold and the wet. If your feet become cold, wet or worse—both, you will be MISERABLE. I recommend treating the shoe with water-proofing spray or rub, which can be found at any shoe store or a camping store. Snow seal is also a great product for this use. It will also increase the life of your shoes.

If you are a dedicated cyclocross racer and will race in every type of weather, then you should definitely have a pair of winter/arctic shoes. This shoe will be a ¾ shoe with a cover to prevent snow from getting inside and a liner for added warmth.

Pedals

Getting in and out of the pedals is VERY important. If you can't get out, you will either crash OR get really good at bunny hopping barriers. If you can't get in, you won't be able to turn the cranks very well. Pedal choice is very important.

One of the best new pedals to emerge, wasn't designed with cyclocross in mind, but tends to work better than most of its predecessors. The Crankbrothers Eggbeater series pedal is light, simple and mud proof. The design is a four-sided entry with such a generous sized cleat trap that mud has no chance of interfering with its

Scott Mares

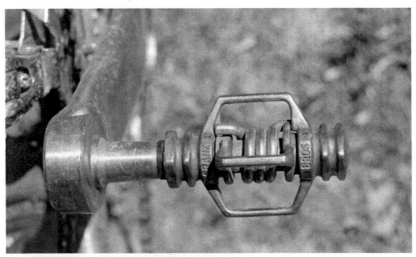

Egg-beater pedals are the way to go.

function. If you get a rock in your shoe, that's a different story.

You can choose a variety of makes and models of the eggbeater to fit your budget. The "Candy" series is the same design, but with an added platform. I would not recommend this pedal for cyclocross because the action is not as positive as the regular eggbeater series. At first look, the Candy would seem like a better pedal because it offers a platform for your foot while the original does not. However, I have found that the eggbeater is actually the better pedal for cyclocross since it allows for entry at any angle. I know more than a few riders that have switched because they were having problems clipping into their candies quickly. The reason is that even though the candy offers a little more of a platform that platform can hinder clicking into the pedal in muddy situations

Clothing

Now, what's in the cyclocrosser's bag? In this section, we will cover the clothing requirements and the tricks of the trade that make preparation and racing easier. Going to a road race requires a minimal amount of clothing. You need a short sleeve jersey, shorts and a light base layer and maybe some arm warmers and a vest. In cyclocross, the temperatures cover a wider range and can be extreme. During the cyclocross season, the weather is starting to change (i.e. It will be 70 degrees one day and a front will move through and the high for the next day will be in the 40s). This means that the cyclocross racer has to have a little more in their bag than the typical road racer.

- Jerseys: Short sleeve, long sleeve and winter

- Jackets: Vest, Wind and winter

- Skin suits: Long sleeve and short sleeve

- Base Layers: Summer, fall and winter base layers

- Knickers: At least one pair, preferably water resistant

- Knee Warmers: At least one pair

- Hats: 3, 1ball cap, 2 fleece

- Shoes: At least one pair for each season (summer, fall and winter)

- Gloves: At least one pair for each season

- Helmets: Two (in case a strap breaks)

- Socks: At least two pairs for each season

- Glasses: Two pair with multiple lenses for changing light conditions

- Embrocations: Warming oils and barrier oils

- Icy Hot patches: Several of varying sizes

- Plastic bags: For putting dirty clothes in

- Towels: One large (in case you need to change in the parking lot) and one medium to dry off

- Cow Bell (Large): You will want one for cheering on other racers.

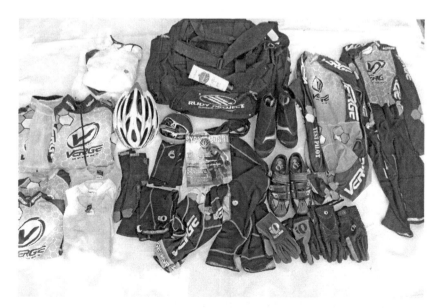

What the typical CX gear bag might contain during mid-season.

Inge Wortman

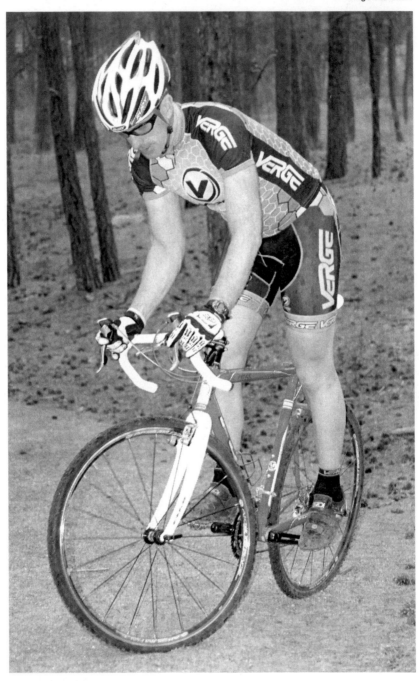

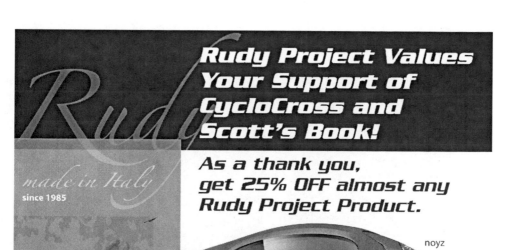
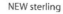
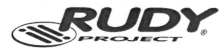

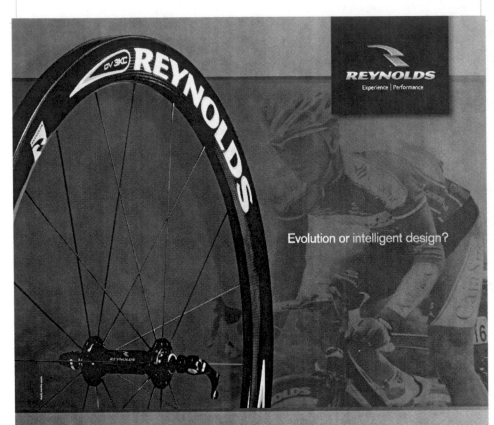

Evolution or intelligent design?

Our carbon clinchers offer the best of both.

In 2003 we introduced the first 100% carbon clincher wheels. Thanks to brilliant engineering and a passionate commitment to carbon technology, our carbon clincher line has evolved into the world's largest. Regardless of rim depth, hub and spoke configuration, weight, or finish, Reynolds carbon clinchers all share something unique. Each is hand-built using our proprietary, advanced carbon layup technology, and one-piece design. The result is enhanced stiffness, reduced weight, superior braking, and unequalled durability.

There's no debate. Reynolds clinchers deliver everything you'd expect from a great carbon wheel. Except the glue. Stop by any Reynolds dealer, and be prepared to experience the ride of your life.™

www.reynoldscycling.com

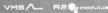

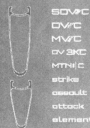

VMS⌒   R2⦿ modulus

SDV/C
DV/C
MV/C
DV 3KC
MTN||C
strike
assault
attack
element

◀ Cutaway view of Reynolds exclusive one piece carbon clincher design.

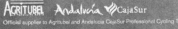

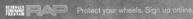

Official supplier to Agritubel and Andalucia CajaSur Professional Cycling Teams

Protect your wheels. Sign up online.

Race Week Routine

Now that you have done all of this work, you're ready to mix it up for real on the cyclocross circuit with your friends. Now is the time to put it all together and develop a race day routine.

Race Week

Four days before the race, gather as much intelligence about the course as possible. If it's in your town, go scope it out and ride it a bit. Get a map of the racecourse and make notes about it. Make sure you have the right tires and gears for the course. Check the weather

Scott Mares

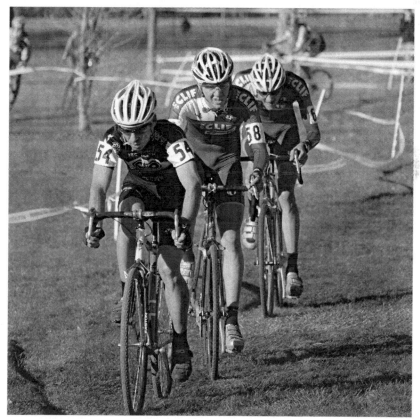

2007 Boulder Cup. Riders are chasing hard.

so you will know what clothing to bring and prepare mentally for the potential conditions. Go over the course in your head and begin preparing mentally for race day.

Check your bike. There are several things to go over now. Do you need new tires? Are you wheels true? When was the last time you replaced your brakes? During a cyclocross race, you do a lot of breaking and your pads can wear out very quickly. Make sure you have an extra set in your toolbox just in case. If you bike needs any maintenance, now is the time to take it to a bike shop.

Two Days before Race

This is your last chance to try anything new like tire pressure or new shifters. Tires should be glued on by now and your bike should be ready to go. Again, check the weather! It can change and so must your strategy and preparation. You may also want to check the promoter's web site to see if there are any changes in the schedule or the course itself..

Day Before

Bike done, spare bike and wheels are ready. Check the weather and get the forecast in that area. If you have to travel you will want this. (do you notice a pattern here?). Have a plan "B" if the weather changes. Check the web site to see if there have been course changes. Some promoters will move the course to a different location or cancel the race if there is really heavy weather. Look at last week's results. Know who your competition is by studying their strengths and weakness. Formulate your race plan and tactics.

Race Day Routine

Get up and check the weather! This will dictate just about everything that you will do and what will happen before, during, and after the race. If you're lucky you can get an hour-by-hour forecast on the temperature and changing weather conditions. Not only will this affect your clothing selection but your tire selection as well. Get there early to register and set up. Go walk the course and watch other people ride the different sections. Take mental notes where the best lines are. After you have walked the course, ride the course. Determine which area is best to ride on for each section and how you plan to attack potentially tough elements of the course. After you have scouted the course, get on the trainer and do your race warm-up. While you are doing your race warm up, go over the course in your head. This will help you to relax tremendously before and during the race. Roll up to the line 5-8 minutes before the start. Make sure to do some stretching and have a friend or team mate take your jacket from you before the start if you are wearing one.

Margaret Fogg

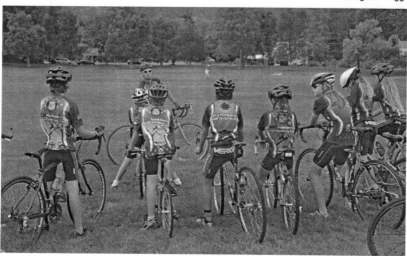

Mudskippers take instruction from Head Coach Dick Elliot at practice.

Post Race

Post race is a very important aspect of the entire routine. You need a cool down and a recovery meal. Your cool down should consist of a 30-minute spin on a trainer or going on a ride on the road for 30 minutes or so. Make sure that you put on **dry** warm clothing for this, meaning you should wear a warm jacket, new dry gloves, dry hat, etc. Following this guideline may not be necessary in mild weather not be that apparent in mild weather but it will be CRITICAL in very cool or cold or wet weather. Make sure that you have a recovery drink with you on your cool down.

Your recovery meal should be eaten right after your cool down. Have a sandwich with some other healthy snacks. Most importantly, make sure you have plenty to drink to re-hydrate.

Post-Race Report

Ok great job on your cyclocross race! Now what happened and what did you learn? One way to make sure you got the most out of your race is to do a post race report. The key to getting the best value out of this exercise is to make it as detailed as possible. I like to have as few parts to the race report as possible and to keep it simple. In the first section, write down the date and time andrace weather conditions. Indicate what you ate before the race and during your warm up.The next section needs to have a few paragraphs about the race itself and should include your start, the middle, and the end of the race. Then draw a map of the race course and make sure you put in turns and geographical features. This would be mud, sand, grass, barriers, run ups, etc. Make sure you draw them in. After you do this, make a column and list the things you did correctly, no matter how small. This is to include that your warm up was good, tire pressure was right on, etc. In the next column, write 3 things that you could improve on or that you wish you had done differently. ONLY write 3. The reason is that any race is a success if you learned something from it.

Tricks and Tips

You know there is nothing like having experience and knowing what works and what doesn't work. In this section, I'll list some tips and tricks that I have picked up over the years that will help you avoid some of the pitfalls you can encounter in cyclocross.

Snow Seal: Treat your shoes with this product when it rains or snows and your feet will stay dry.

RainX Wipes: Wipe some RainX on your glasses so they will not hold on to the water or the mud that gets kicked up in a race. Wipe your frame down with it and you will notice that your frame will shed mud more easily.

Reverse Your Brakes: Why? If your rear brake is on the left you can control your speed into the barrier without having the bike flip. Having the front brake on the left can cause the bike to endo (flip over and crash), if you try to control the speed into a barrier.

Big (one gallon) Zip Loc Bags: Have one for gloves, one for base layers and so on. This way you will not lose an item on the bottom of your duffle bag and you will be able to have everything where you can find it.

WD40: Spraying WD40 will prevent mud build up.

ArmorAll: Spray on the frame to help keep off the build up and mud and in most cases the mud will shed off the bike more easily.

Antifreeze: Have a small spray bottle of antifreeze and spray the drive train to prevent icing and freezing.

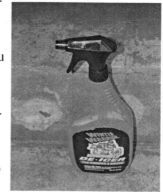

Spoke Treatment: Treat the spokes with WD40/Pam or RainX. This way you won't have muddy spokes in a race.

Rim treatment: If you have an aero deep section rim, treat the non-break surface so you do not carry any extra mud around.

Pam: This is another favorite to keep the frame mud free.

Support Staff (i.e. good buddy or family member): Having someone to take your jacket from you at the start line just before the start of the race is just good common sense.

Identical Bikes: Having a spare bike is very important. Having the bike set up identically is also just as important.

Separate Race Clothing: Go warm up in cycling clothing and just before your final prep, change into some nice clean and dry clothing. Staying warm and dry is very important. Being cold and wet is BAD. Change your shoes if you need to as well.

Icy Hot Patches: Icy hot makes patches that stick to you and have warming lotion. If you apply the patch to the center of your back, it will help keep you warm. You can apply them to other areas as well. I'm a big fan of putting them on my knees.

Vaseline: This is a good one for a water barrier. It's not just for

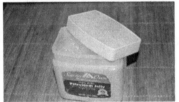

your lips! You can put it on your legs. This will keep you dry. It's also used to put on your cycling pad to keep you from chafing.

Bike Stand: If you don't have a mechanic to hand you a bike in the pit, you will need a bike stand so you won't have to lay your spare bike on the ground. Set up the bike stand in the pit so you will be ready to grab it and go. There are a few bike stands on the market that are designed to make it easy to quickly grab your bike and get back out there. Make sure you put your name and phone number on the stand in case someone takes it from the pit by mistake.

Safety Pins: If you race in Europe, they don't furnish pins with your number like we do here in the US. Got skinny legs? Safety pin your knee warmers to the bottom of your shorts to prevent them ending up around you ankles They will keep them from falling down around your ankles.

Clear Shower Cap: A clear shower cap fits over your helmet and keeps your head warm and dry. (Remember, dry is good!)

Clear Packing Tape: Place clear packing tape over the vents of your helmet to prevent snow and rain from coming in and getting your head wet..You can also use on your the packing tape on your chain stay to protect your frame from chain slap.

Embrodication: The weather can vary and you need protection for your skin in the cold and wet. There are several types out there that will create that vapor barrier on your skin and keep you warm.

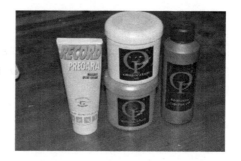

Strength and Core Conditioning for Cyclocross "CX" Racing

By Scott Hackett C.S.C.S.
dirtcoach@gmail.com

Why is it Important?

The discipline of Cyclocross "CX" racing places a wide range of demands on the neuromuscular system of the rider, more so than most other forms of bicycle racing. From sprinting at the start for position, pushing a big gear on the flats, accelerating out of corners,

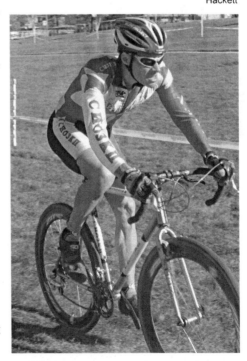

Hackett

dismounts and remounts at 20 mph, bounding over barriers, lifting and carries of the bike up hills and stairs, slugging through mud snow and sand, then sprinting for the win. Besides the specific cyclocross skill development and on bike energy system development outlined within this manual there is one area of importance that most cyclists of any discipline have given little attention to, that is strength and core training.

While no one can dispute that a stronger athlete is a better athlete and that it is true for any cyclist as well. There is also undeniable proof that strength-training is the most effec-

Frank Hibbits turns on the afterburners

tive way to become stronger athlete. Still there are detractors of strength training for endurance athletes', these naysayers point out two main concerns for both the recreational and elite cyclist, he first concern is the increased muscle mass will not help the cyclist in most areas especially if climbing is important, the second concern is that time spent strength training takes time away from actual cycling. Most often when the cyclist does strength train it is undertaken in a haphazard manner with little thought and planning as to how it will impact the short term and long term performance positive or negative. What is needed is for the coach or trainer and athlete is to implement an effective intergraded periodized strength plan for optimal performance improvements. Periodization is commonly and effectively utilized for endurance training though rarely is a perodized core and strength plan intergraded within the main training plan for endurance sport athletes.

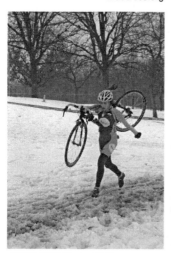

Mudcross.org

2007 WI State CX Championships, Hales Corner, Wisconsin

The cyclocross racer or any endurance athlete should understand the distinct differences of strength training for specific performance adaptations verses the typical so called fitness and body building type weight training. These types of weight training are for primarily appearance purposes were muscle hypertrophy and fat loss is usually the objective and do little to improve or actually harm an athlete's performance. To further confuse those looking for improved endurance performance there is Olympic weight lifting and power lifting. All of these forms of weight lifting have been used for endurance sports with very disappointing results by the inexperienced and uneducated in development and implementation of performance orientated functional strength and core training programs. Since all these types of weight training are ineffective for endurance athletes' detractors contend that strength training does not have any benefits for the cyclist.

Contrary to previously discussed ineffective weight-training regimes, the benefits' of an effective and functional strength and core-conditioning program where the objective is increased performance by improved neuromuscular function, not just because the muscles are bigger.

So what is an effective and functional strength-training program for a cyclocross racer like and how should one integrate into their training you may ask? To answer those questions lets look at what it means to be a stronger cyclocross racer then define the performance objectives and benefits of an effective strength training program for the cyclocross racer. To be a stronger cyclocross racer means to be able effectively transfer power from one leg to the other while cycling, dismounting, running while shouldering or pushing the bike, running over barriers up stairs, remounting while decelerating as little as possible, re-acceleration from low speed and a strong sprint for position or finish.

Performance objectives and benefits of an effective strength and core-training program.

The list below is not in any particular order of importance as that differs from athlete to athlete are:

- Decreased neuromuscular inhibition leading to increased force production.

- Limit overall muscular hypertrophy.

- Increase short-term muscular endurance for increased sprinting ability.

- Increased medium to long-term muscular endurance when pushing a big gear on the flats.

- Increased acceleration power for starts, out of corners or launching an attack.

- Increased muscular elasticity for dismounts and remounts and running over barriers.

- Both dynamic and static stability of the core musculature for lifting and carries of the bike up hills and stairs.

- Correcting muscular imbalances.

- Injury prevention.

- Increased ability to withstand higher training loads.

- More favorable body composition.

Now that we have defined the objectives and benefits of an effective functional core and strength training program, what exactly is functional strength and core training anyway? Lets start at the actual definition of functional.

Func.tion.al 1. capable of operating or functioning 2. having or serving a utilitarian purpose; capable of serving the purpose for which it was designed. *(Webster's Encyclopedia Unabridged Dictionary of the English Language, 2nd Edition, 1996)*

The general characteristics of a functional exercise for the cyclocross rider are:

- Improves relevant biomotor abilities for the primary sport being cyclocross

- General motor program compatibility for the primary sport being cyclocross

- Improves and or maintenance righting and equilibrium reflexes for both cycling and running with carrying a bicycle over barriers up and down hills

- Maintenance of your Center of Gravity on your own base of support

- Static postural component

- Dynamic postural component

- Open/Closed Chain compatibility

As Gray Cook (a leading expert in the rehabilitative, strength and conditioning field) states that "Core training can be just another fad or it can be a scientifically-based methodology that involves a functional and progressive approach to movement re-education and performance enhancement." The truth is most fitness enthusiasts to professional athletes still believe the abdominals and primarily the rectus abdominus (the six pack muscles) is your core. This being the case core training for most still differs little than from 20 years ago were crunches and side bends made up the majority of the time spent so called core training. When you understand that the core is all the muscles between your limbs, not just the abdominals,

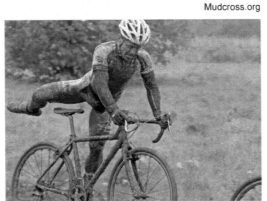
Mudcross.org

2006 Trash Dash Cyclocross, Whitewater, Wisconsin. A muddy rider removing his bike.

these include the back muscles deep and superficial, hip flexors, gluteus muscles and of course your deep and superficial abdominals. Cook explains function within human movement this way. "You must understand that the brain recognizes movement patterns and not simply muscle groups. Yet, many professionals are still stuck in isolation training or muscle group training. Understanding movement patterns is a little more in-depth and complicated than simply understanding muscle groups. You also need to understand that the most fundamental activities of the human body revolve around simple and basic movements of running and climbing. Running demands that a spine be stable and transfer energy from one leg to the other as well as deal with the counterbalance movement of the arms as they swing, whereas climbing requires that the spine be mobile, adaptable and dynamic. These are two very fundamental movements of the human body, and yet they contrast each other in their demands of the core."

Cyclocross racing is no different in the need to transfer muscular power from one leg to the other, but also must support the upper body in a semi-seated position that can be either static or dynamic that creates greater stresses on the lumbar spine than running. No wonder many cyclists have sore and stiff backs or worse develop back injuries from cycling. It is easy to spot a cyclist with poor core stability and dynamic strength as they pedal they weave from side to side since their weak cores are allowing their upper body to sway and bob causing the handle bars to move wasting a significant amount energy in the process. A mobile, adaptable and dynamic spine is also important for cyclocross especially when dismounting, re-mounting and carries common in cyclocross racing. Effective core and strength training exercises for cyclocross racing should focus on stability and dynamic movement of the core musculature, exercises that are also self supported, multi joint single leg that reinforce movement patterns within cyclocross racing and develop muscular strength and power through decreased neuromuscular inhibition without unwanted hypertrophy.

Modalities and Exercises?

Now that you have a greater understanding of the true demands of cyclocross racing on the neuromuscular system, the objectives and benefits of core and strength training. What actually functional core and strength training is and the characteristics of strength and core exercises for cyclocross racing. We are getting closer to putting the program together though within the program there are six training modalities with objectives and benefits within the whole program that must first be understood. The first three modalities (Movement Preparation, Prehabilitation and Physioball) I consider the power trio the fundamental core of the whole program without them all other modalities are substantially less effective. Implementing these simple routines will improve nearly every aspect of your performance and daily living and are of the highest priority within the programs I design.

Movement Preparation

Movement preparation is a routine of dynamic exercise movements that is far superior to the traditional warm up and pre-exercise stretching as the routine prepares the body for higher intensity movement be it cycling, running, strength training or gardening. Movement preparation increases the heart rate, blood blow to the muscles, raises the core temperature and will also improve the function of the neuromuscular system. There are two movement prep routines one for Strength Training and Cycling Activities and another for Running, Elasticity, Plyometric, Cyclocross Drills and Skills.

Prehabilitation (Prehab)

Most athletes' are familiar with rehabilitation, whereas prehabilitation is a proactive approach to training instead of waiting for an injury to occur that was almost certainly preventable. Common injured areas such as the shoulders, hips, and low back are the primary focus. To prevent injuries and surgeries that would have required rehabilitation, or rehab, Prehab is any athletes' best friend.

Physioball (PB)

Also known as the Stability Ball or Swiss Ball, used in clinical rehabilitation for over 30 years. Due to their effectiveness physioballs have recently become popular as a training aid in developing balance and dynamic core strength. The exercises described are a key component within this program and can be done throughout the year.

The next two training modalities (Elasticity/Reactivity and Strength) are dynamic duo of the complete program outlined within this chapter. By intergrading either Elasticity or Strength into you training program will result increased cyclocross performance, but combining the two may be the knock out punch to your competition. Within the programs for the endurance athletes I train and coach these two have significant impact of the athletes' conditioning profile though they do have a lower priority of importance compared to the previous power trio.

Elasticity / Reactivity

More commonly referred to as plyometrics that can best be described as "explosive-reactive" power training. This type of training involves powerful muscular contractions in response to a rapid stretching of the involved musculature. These powerful contractions are not a pure muscular they have a high degree of central nervous system involvement. Elasticity and reactivity exercises are a combination of an involuntary reflex (a neural event), which is then followed by a fast voluntary muscular contraction.

Strength

The strength routine is comprised of exercises that fulfill the components of a functional strength program previously discussed, those being: Comparable Reflex Profile (Righting and Equilibrium reflexes), Maintenance of your Center of Gravity over your own base of support, Static postural component, Dynamic postural component, Generalized motor program compatibility, Open/Closed chain compatibility, Improves the relevant biomotor abilities for the primary sport or activity training for being Cyclocross.

For the purposes of this manual I'm not going into great detail of the final modality of Regeneration, but to provide a short synopsis of the basic information that can be downloaded in detail by visiting Coach Scott Hackett on the web at ww.JDSsportcoaching.com

Regeneration

The final modality (Regeneration) is often the unsung hero or invisible man of most training programs. That is that athletes and trainers alike do not give much credit to the role regeneration has in an athletes training program. Even worse is when the invisible man approach is used, were no real attention in the way of planning for it within the training plan let alone as to ways to improve your recovery through other methods. Although the intensity of training is important, another key factor is the type of training performed has on recovery. For example, exercises that have a higher eccentric component, like dismounts to clear a barrier and the elasticity, reactivity exercises discussed within this chapter both would require more recovery time than say a simple run or bike ride. It is important to note that recovery is more effective if a variety of techniques are used rather than just a single method alone. For the cyclist this single method has usually been in the form of a recovery spin though usually I find most endurance athletes do these recovery workouts at to high of an intensity and duration to be really considered active recovery.

A short list of effective methods to increase recovery:

- Sleep the main physiological means of restoration.

- Food

- Kino therapy (Active Recovery and Movement Therapy)

- Myofascial Release Techniques (Massage, Foam Rolling and Stretching)

- Hydrotherapy (Hot and Cold Showers)

- Electro Muscle Stimulation and Ultrasound

- Mental Relaxation

- Chemotherapy (Nutritional Supplementation)

The two regeneration modes discussed here are Foam Rolling and Stretching in the form of what is called Active-Isolated Stretching. I suggest performing both AIS and Foam Rolling later in the evening during the hour going to sleep for the night as this really helps you relax and stimulates the body's healing response while the muscles are in a relaxed and lengthened state further enhancing recovery.

Foam Rolling

A foam roller is simply a cylindrical piece of hard-celled foam, like a swimming pool noodle, but more dense and larger in diameter. The application techniques for foam rolling are simple, based on an acupressure concept, in

which pressure is placed on specific surfaces of the body
and for self-massage. The idea is to allow athletes to apply
pressure to injury-prone areas themselves; essentially
foam rollers can be used as the poor man's massage therapist. A foam rolling session is not as thorough as a good
deep tissue massage they provide effective soft tissue
work to the masses for $20 - $50 and can be used over and
over that will aid in injury prevention and performance
enhancement.

Active-Isolated Stretching

What differentiates Active-Isolated Stretching (AIS) also
called "contract–relax." from the more common static
stretching is that this method requires that you place the
muscle to be stretched under tension and then activate it
against isometric (immovable) resistance for five seconds
by contracting the apposing muscle group, followed immediately by five seconds of relaxed lengthening, then return-
ing to the starting position. Many of the stretches are facili-
tated by using your own hands, a partner, a device such as a
rope, my favorite an extra heavy theraband or physioball to
gently enhance the stretch and to maintain alignment.

Below are the exercises and photo for each of the first five modalities that comprise the sample program.

Movement Prep Routine A for Strength Training and Cycling Activities

Forward Lunge/Forearm-to-Instep *

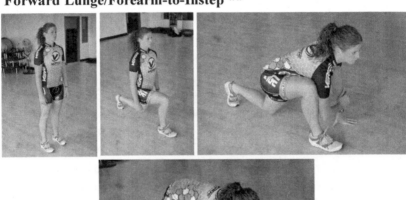

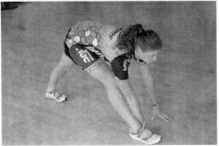

Backward Lunge with a Twist *

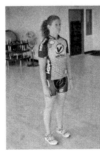
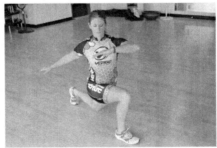

Hand Walk Forward and Backwards **

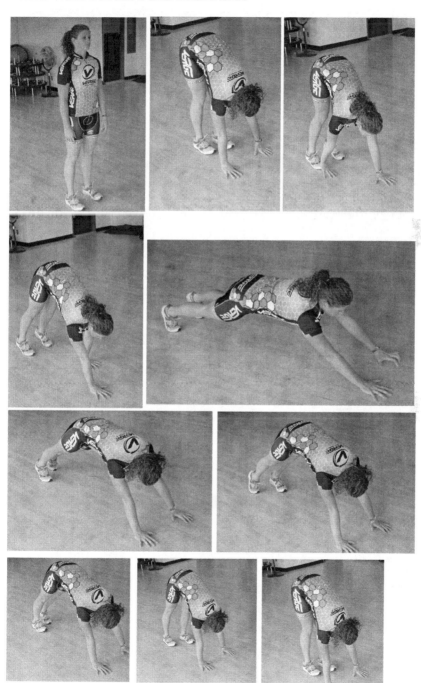

Hip Cross Over

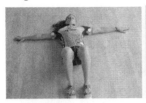 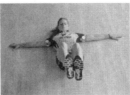 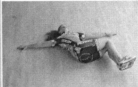

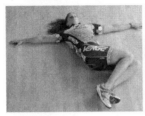 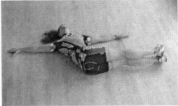

Scorpion

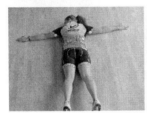 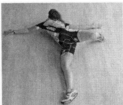

Lateral Lunge

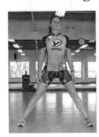 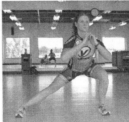 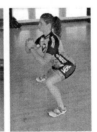

Sumo Squat-to-Stand

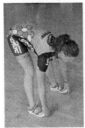 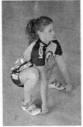

Inverted Hamstring **

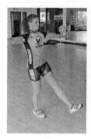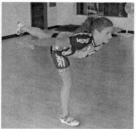

<u>Movement Prep Routine B for Running, Elasticity / Reactivity CX Drills and Skills</u>

Include above exercises from Routine A with **

High Knee Walk

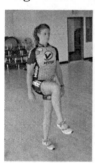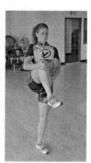

Heel Up

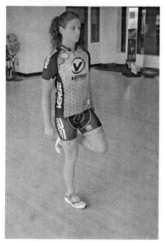

Straight Leg Dead Lift Walk

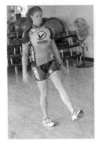 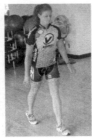 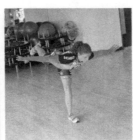

High Knee Skip

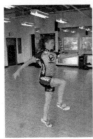 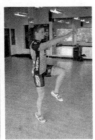

Straight Leg Skip   ### Back Peddle

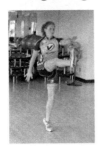   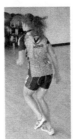 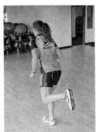

Backward Run

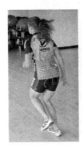 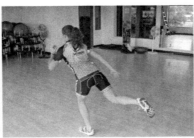

Prehabilitation (Prehab)

Abs and Low back
Prone Bridging

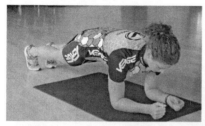 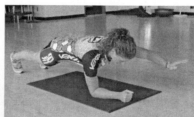

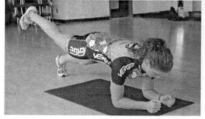 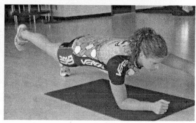

Side Bridging

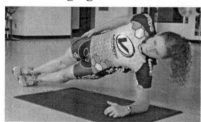 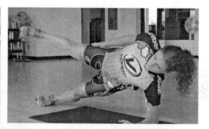

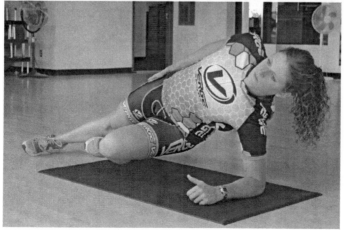

Supine Draw-In with Hip Flexion
(Progression to Feet Supported to unsupported)

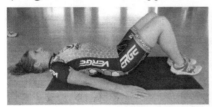 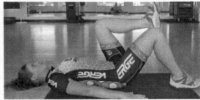

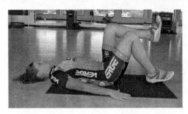

Supine Draw-In with Hip Flexion and Extension
(Progression to Dead Bug)

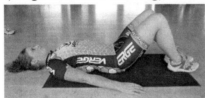 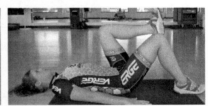

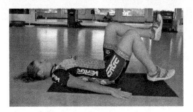

Quadruped Hip Extension
(Progression)

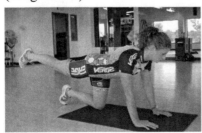 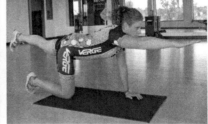

Shoulders
PB T, Y, W, L

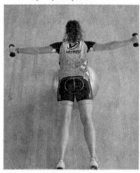 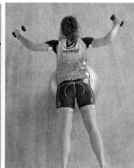 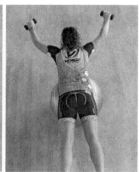

Overhead Reach Against Wall

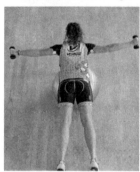 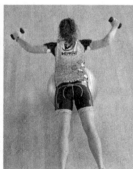 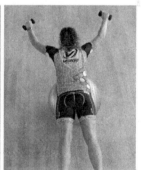

Hips and Glutes
Glute Bridging (Progression to Single Leg)

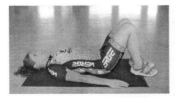
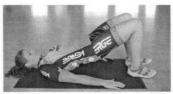

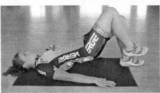
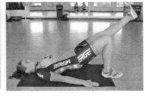

Hip Adduction

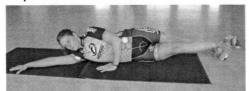

Hip Abduction

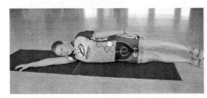
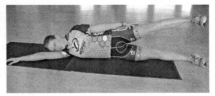

Hip Circles

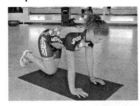
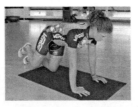

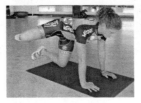
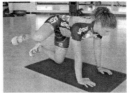

<u>Physioball</u>

PB Push Ups

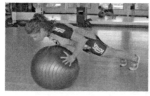 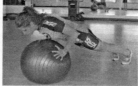

Lateral Roll

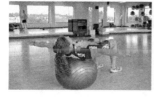 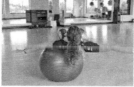

Russian Twist

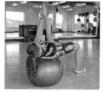 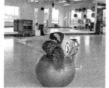

Prone Knee Tucks

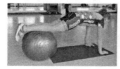 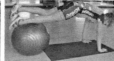 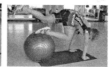

Reverse Crunch

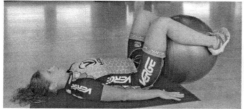 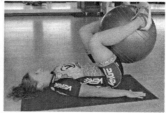

<u>Strength</u>

Split Squat
(Progression to Rear Leg Elevated)

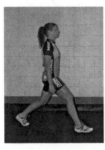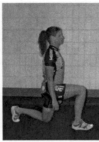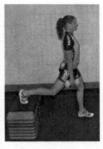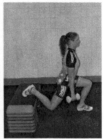

Alternating DB Chest Press w/ arm Drive

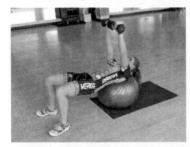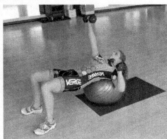

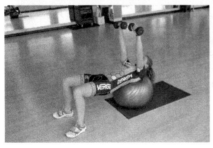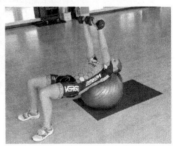

Alternating DB Chest Press Plus

Bench Step Up w/ DB Curl Nieder Press

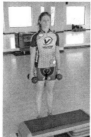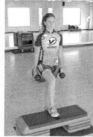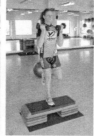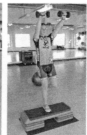

Romanian Dead Lift (modified straight leg)

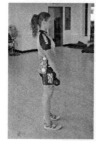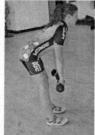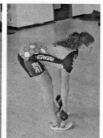

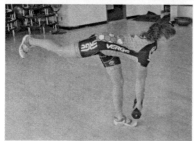

One Arm One Leg Squat Row

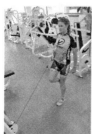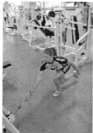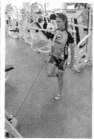

Lunge w/ Bilateral Cable/ Bungee Arm Drive

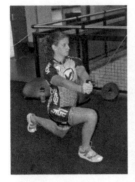 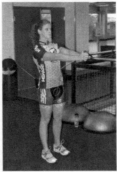

Cable Lifting

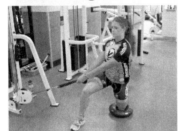 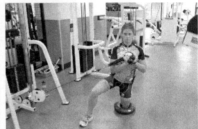

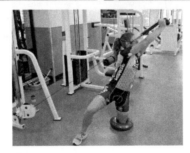

Cable Chopping

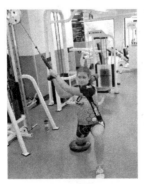 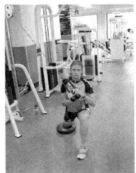 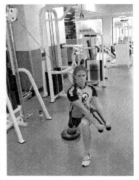

Elasticity and Reactivity

Power Skip

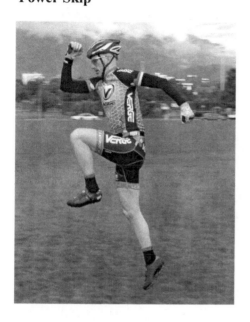

Squat Jump 1 and10's

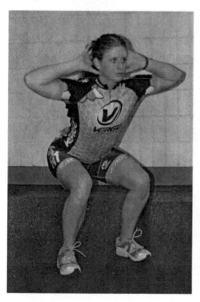 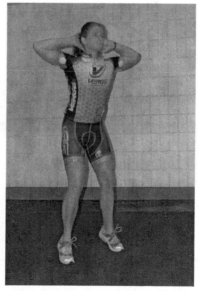

One Leg Jump
(Progression to box)

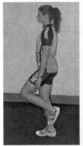 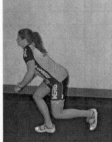 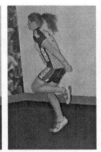 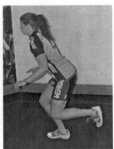

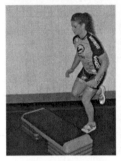 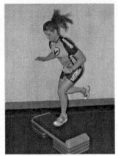

Split Squat Jump

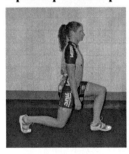 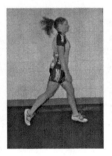 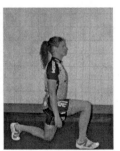

Lateral Bound
(Progression to Continuous)

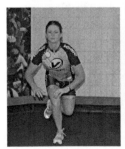 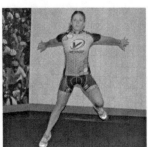 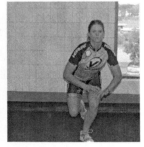

Section Three Putting it all Together

By Scott Hackett C.S.C.S.
Associate Coach JDSsportcoaching LLC

Putting it all together

The program outlined is more than just core and strength training, but a complete system to help your perform better while on the bike and in your daily life. Each daily routine is comprised of different sub-routines from the modalities and exercise outlined in Sections One and Two. As any well thought out periodized training plan this plan changes through out the training year and training cycles. This system allows for development of specific physical abilities during one training phase while maintaining others. For most people even full time elite athletes this is a more practical way to get all components of a compressive training program done with consistency being the most important aspect of any training program. In fact doing everything in a comprehensive training program everyday isn't practical or even the optimal situation for increased performance and your health. The program is designed utilizing one to six sub routines that comprise the daily routine. There will be times that your will not be able to get in everything that I have suggested for your training plan, don't stress out about it, it is better to do one or a couple of the scheduled activities very well than a half hearted attempt at all of them.

An Important detail to note: The following sample plan is for one macro-cycle or training period (Peak to Competitive Maintenance) of a complete periodized plan that can be implemented during the Peak through the Competitive periods of the cyclocross season. For a downloadable package or CD with larger pictures of the exercises and directions on how to perform the exercise movements or complete plan with customized training logs visit Coach Scott Hackett on the web at www.JDSsportcoaching.com

The Workout Sub Routines

Movement Prep A		
Exercise	**Sets**	**Reps**
Forward Lunge/Forearm-to-Instep	1	8 to 15
Backward Lunge with a Twist	1	6 to 12, each side
Hand Walk Forward and Backwards	1	8 to 12
Hip Cross Over	1	6 to 12, each side
Scorpion	1	6 to 12, each side
Lateral Lunge	1	6 to 12, each side
Sumo Squat-to-Stand	1	6 to 12, each sid
Inverted Hamstring	1	8 to 12

Movement Prep B		
Exercise	**Sets**	**Reps / Distance**
Forward Lunge/Forearm-to-Instep	1	6 to 10
Backward Lunge with a Twist	1	6 to 12, each side
Hand Walk Forward	1	6 to 10
High Knee Walk	1	20 meters
Heel Up	1	20 meters
Straight Leg Deed Lift Walk	1	20 meters
High Knee Skip	1 to 2	20 meters
Straight Leg Skip	1 to 2	20 meters
Back Peddle	1 to 2	20 meters
Backward Run	1 to 2	20 meters

Prehab Abs and Low Ba			
Excercise	**Sets**	**Reps**	**Hold Time**
Prone Bridging (Progression)	1 to 2	6 to 10	30 to 90
Side Bridging (Progression)	1 to 2	6 to 10	15 to 60
Supine Draw-In w/ Hip Flexion (Progress to Feet Unsupported)	1 to 2	6 to 10	30 to 90 seconds
Or Supine Draw-In w/Hip Fexion to Extension (progress to Dead	1 to 2	6 to 10	30 to 90 seconds
Quadruped Hip Extension (Progression to Physioball)	1 to 2	6 to 10	30 to 90 seconds

Prehab Shoulders			
Excercise	**Sets**	**Reps**	**Hold Time**
T	1 to 2	8 to 15	Pause 5 seconds
Y			
W			
L (Progression to Physioball)			
Overhead Reach Against the Wall	2 to 4	6 to 10	Pause 5 seconds

Prehab Hips and Glutes			
Excercise	**Sets**	**Reps**	**Hold Time**
Glute Bridging (Progression to	1 to 2	8 to 15	3 to 10 seconds Pause
Hip Adduction	1 to 2	10 to 15	Pause 5 seconds
Hip Adduction	1 to 2	10 to 15	Pause 5 seconds
Hip Circles (Each	1	10 to 15	
Overhead Reach	2 to 4	6 to 10	Pause 5 seconds

Physioball		
Exercise	**Sets**	**Reps**
PB Push Ups	1 to 2	8 to 15
Advanced Combine with Knee Tucks	2 to 3	Max Reps
Lateral Roll	1 to 2	10 to 15
Russian Twist - perfect form, start holding weight	2	15
Prone Knee Tucks - perfect form, start	2	15
Reverse Crunch	1 to 2	10 to 15
PB Pulsing	1 to 2	10 to 30 seconds

Strength			
Excercise	**Sets**	**Reps**	**% of 1RM**
Split Squat			
(Progression to Rear Leg Elevated)	1 to 2	10 to 20	55 to 75%
Alternating DB Chest Press Plus	1 to 2	10 to 20	55 to 75%
Or Alternating DB Chest Press w/ arm Drive	1 to 2	10 to 20	55 to 75%
Bench Step Up w/ DB Curl Nieder Press	1 to 2	10 to 20	55 to 75%
Romanian Dead Lift		1 to 2	10 to 20
One Arm One Leg Squat Row	1 to 2	10 to 20	55 to 75%
Cable Chopping	1 to 2	10 to 20	55 to 75%
Lunge w/ Bilateral Arm Drive	1 to 2	10 to 20	55 to 75%
Cable Lifting	1 to 2	10 to 20	55 to 75%

For those less experienced with strength training (less than three solid years) the strength movements can be performed as a circuit for higher reps 15 to 20 at 55-65% of 1RM one after another with 30 to 45 seconds of recovery before moving on to the next movement.

For those with more experience, the routine can also be performed as Super Sets. Supper Sets are two exercises performed one after another with 20 to 30 seconds of recovery between each exercise for reps of 10 to 15 at 65-75% of 1RM and a two minute recovery before the next set or Super Set is performed.

Whether experienced or not, I also combine several of the Physioball exercises into the Strength routines. This a great time saving and effective alternative.

Elasticity and Reactivity		
Recommended 3 exercises are chosen per workout		
Exercise	**Sets**	**Reps** /
Power Skip	2 to 4	20 to 40 meters
Squat Jump	1 to 3	4 to 10
Advanced Squat Jump	1	10
One Leg Jump (Progression to box)	1 to 3	4 to 10 each leg
Split Squat Jump Switch	1 to 3	4 to 10
Lateral Bound (Progression to Continuous)	1 to 3	E4 to 10

Weekly Schedule For a Pre-Competitive Peak or a Non Race Week

Monday	
EST: Trainer/Rollers Spin 30-40 minutes Intensity: Zone 1	
Core Strength Sub Routine	**Time to Complete**
Movement Prep A	8 minutes
Prehab: Shoulder	5 minutes
Prehab: Hips Glutes	5 minutes
Regeneration: Foam Roller	8-15 minutes
Regeneration: AIS	8-10 minutes

Tuesday
EST: Ride 70 to 100 minutes Intensity: VO$_2$ Intervals: one to two sets of three to eight reps CX Skills: 20-30 minutes at half-speed aspart of warm up/warm down of bike workout Advanced Riders combine Dis/Re-Mounts, Bike Hill Carries with Intervals

Core Strength Sub Routine	Time to Complete
Prehab: Core	8 minutes
Movement Prep B	12 minutes
Elasticity and Reactivity	7 minutes (one set)
Strength	20 minutes

I have found over the years that it is much more effective to combine on the same day intense intervals (VO$_2$s, Hill Sprints, Sprints) with strength training this is because the energy systems and recovery periods are similar for both.

Rather than what is usually done of hard intervals one day followed by strength training the next or the other way around, with this arrangement, the second training day's objectives are always compromised and recovery will be two to three times longer.

Wednesday
EST: Ride 90 to 180 minutes Intensity: Zone 2 Six 20 second acceleration spin-ups (undergeared)

Core Strength Sub Routine	Time to Complete
Movement Prep A	8 minutes
Regeneration: Foam Roller	8-15 minutes
Regeneration: AIS	8-10 minutes

Thursday

EST: Run 20 to 30 minutes, Hilly Route
Intensity Zone: 2 to 3
Bike 40 to 90 minutes Flat to Rolling
Intensity Zone 2 with four to eight, 30 to 40 second Hill Sprints

Core Strength Sub Routine	Time to Complete
Movement Prep B	12 minutes
Elasticity and Reactivity	12 minutes (two to three sets)
Physioball	10 minutes
Regeneration: Foam Roller	8-15 minutes

Friday

EST: Day Off

Core Strength Sub Routine	Time to Complete
Movement Prep A	8 minutes
Regeneration: Foam Roller	8-15 minutes
Regeneration: AIS	8-10 minutes

Saturday

EST: Ride 90 to 120 minutes
Intensity Zone: Mixed with VO_2 Intervals one set of two to four reps
Threshold Intervals two to three reps of 8 to 12 minutes each
CX Skills: 20 to 30 minutes at half to full speed as part of warm up / warm down of bike workout.
Advanced Riders combine Dis/Re-Mounts, Bike Hill Carries in the early stage of threshold Intervals

Core Strength Sub Routine	Time to Complete
Movement Prep B	8 minutes
Elasticity and Reactivity	12 to 15 minutes (two to three sets)
Strength	20 minutes
Regeneration: AIS	8 to 10 minutes

Sunday

EST: Ride 150 to 240 minutes
Intensity Zone: 2, 3-4 Tempo
Strength Endurance with six, 20 sec acceleration spin-ups (undergeared)
Run 15 to 30 minutes
Intensity Zone: 2 to 3
Option as second workout four to five hours later

Core Strength Sub Routine	Time to Complete
Movement Prep A	8 minutes
Regeneration: AIS	8 to 10 minutes
Option:	
Regeneration: Foam Roller	8 to 15 minutes

Weekly Schedule For a One Race Week

Monday

EST: Trainer/Rollers Spin 30 to 40 minutes
Intensity Zone: 1

Core Strength Sub Routine	Time to Complete
Movement Prep A	8 minutes
Prehab: Shoulder	5 minutes
Prehab: Hips Glutes	5 minutes
Regeneration: Foam Roller	8 to 15 minutes
Regeneration: AIS	8 to 10 minutes

Tuesday

EST: Ride 70-100 minutes
Intensity VO_2 Intervals 1 set of three to eight reps
CX Skills: 10 to 20 minutes at half to thre-quarter speed as part of warm up /
warm down of bike workout. Advanced Riders combine Dis/Re-Mounts, Bike
Hill Carries with Intervals

Core Strength Sub Routine	Time to Complete
Prehab: Core	8 minutes
Movement Prep B	12 minutes
Strength	20 minutes

Wednesday

EST: Ride 70 to 150 minutes
Intensity Zone: 2
Six, 20 second acceleration spin-ups (undergeared)

Core Strength Sub Routine	Time to Complete
Movement Prep A	8 minutes
Regeneration: Foam Roller	8 to 15 minutes
Strength	8 to 10 minutes

Thursday

EST: Bike 40 to 90 minutes Flat to Rolling
Intensity Zone: 2 to 3
Four to eight, 30 to 40 second Hill Sprints
CX Skills: 30 to 40 minutes at half to full speed
Bike Hill carries of 20 to 30 seconds are optional substitution for bike Hill sprints
or mix

Core Strength Sub Routine	Time to Complete
Movement Prep B	12 minutes
Elasticity and Reactivity	10 minutes (two to three sets)
Physioball	10 minutes
Regeneration: Foam Roller	8 to 15 minutes

Friday

EST: Day Off	Day Off
Core Strength Sub Routine	**Time to Complete**
Movement Prep A	8 minutes
Regeneration: Foam Roller	8 to 15 minutes
Regeneration: AIS	8 to 10 minutes

Saturday

EST: Ride 40-60 mins
Intensity Zone: 2 with one set of two VO2 intervals two minutes each with five
minutes of complete recovery between them

Core Strength Sub Routine	Time to Complete
Movement Prep B	8 minutes
Regeneration: AIS	8 to 10 minutes

Sunday	
EST: Warm Up and Race Post Race: Spin 20 to 60 minutes Intensity Zone: 1 to 2	
Core Strength Sub Routine	**Time to Complete**
Movement Prep A	8 minutes
Regeneration: AIS	8 to 10 minutes
Regeneration: Foam Roller	8 to 15 minutes

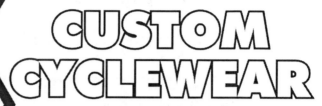

CUSTOM CYCLEWEAR

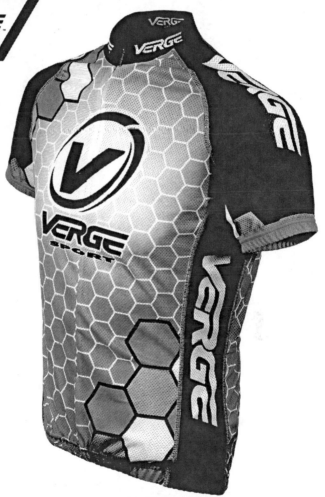

1-800-536-0160
VERGESPORT.COM

The Leader in American Cyclo-Cross since 1994

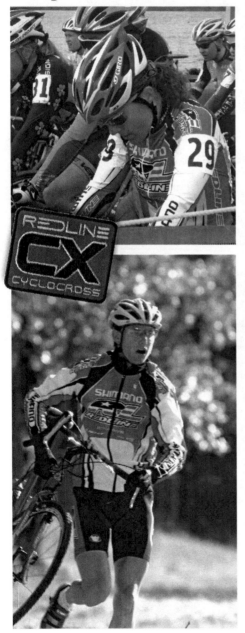

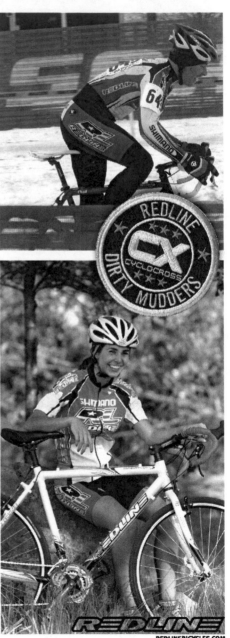

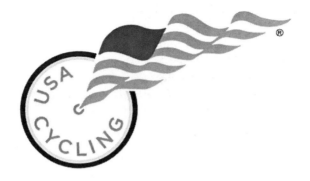

Cyclocross Rules

Reprinted with permission from USA Cycling.

5. Cyclocross

5A. Course and obstacles

5A1. The course shall be held over varying terrain including roads, country or forest paths, and open terrain alternating in such a way as to ensure changes in the pace of the race and allow the riders to recuperate after difficult sections.

5A2. The course shall be rideable in all conditions, regardless of the weather. Clay or easily flooded areas, such as fields, should be avoided.

5A3. The course shall form a closed circuit of a minimum length of 2.5 km and maximum 3.5 km, of which at least 90% shall be rideable (exceptions to this rule may be requested through the CEO or his designee).

5A4. Over its full length, the course shall be a minimum of 3 meters wide and be well marked and protected. The use of dangerous elements, such as wires (barbed or not), and sharp or uncapped metal poles shall be forbidden. Furthermore, the course shall not be placed near any object that could constitute a danger for riders (exceptions to the minimum width rule may be requested through the CEO or his designee).

5A5. An assembly point for starters (roll-call zone) shall be provided and marked off behind the starting line. For championships and other major events eight lanes with a width of 75 cm and a length of 10 meters shall be marked off at the start line to facilitate organizing the riders into starting order.

5A6. The starting stretch shall be a minimum of 200 meters in length and at least 6 meters wide to allow the field to string out properly. It shall be as straight as possible and not downhill. The first narrowing or obstacle after the starting stretch may not be abrupt but shall allow all the riders to pass easily.

5A7. The finishing stretch shall be a straight line. It shall have a minimum length of 100 meters and a minimum width of 6 meters for championships, 4 meters for other events (6 meters is recommended). It shall be flat or uphill.

5A8. The starting and finishing stretches shall be free of obstacles.

5A9. The course shall include a maximum of 6 obstacles (temporary barriers or terrain) designed to oblige (not require) riders to dismount their bike. The length of an obstacle should not be longer than 80 meters. The total length of obstacles may not exceed 10% of the course distance.

5A10. The course may *include a single section* of temporary artificial *barriers. This shall consist of two barriers of wooden or other non-metallic material, standing vertically, 40cm tall, 4 meters apart, and taking up the full width of the race course. The surfaces of the barriers must have no gaps from the top to the ground. Barriers may be placed on flat or uphill terrain; downhill barriers are expressly forbidden.*

5A11. Races which are not UCI events, national championships, or used to qualify riders for national teams or international competition may have two additional sets of temporary artificial barriers (3 total). The barriers must meet the specifications in 5A10 and the total number of obstacles may not exceed 6. The addition of additional temporary barriers should be done only in unusual circumstances (e.g. local tradition at a particular event or the lack of suitable terrain)

5A12. The course may cross bridges or footbridges provided that they are a minimum of 3 meters wide and that there is a guard rail on both sides. A non-slip surface (carpet, wire mesh, or special anti-slip paint) shall be used on bridges and footbridges. A separate footbridge shall be provided for spectators.

5A13. No acrobatics on the part of the riders shall be required to overcome obstacles.

5A14. Having consulted the Organizer, the Chief Referee may decide that artificial obstacles shall be removed if the circuit is unusually slippery.

5A15. For championship events, up to 5 races may be run per day over the same course.

5B. Equipment pits

5B1. An equipment pit is the part of the circuit where riders can change wheels or bicycles. Wheels or bicycles may only be changed in an official equipment pit.

5B2. Two equipment pits shall be located around the course, in agreement with the Chief Referee, in places where speeds are not high but not on stony, gravel, or downhill stretches. They shall be straight and free of obstacles. If, during each lap, the course passes two points sufficiently close to each other, just one pit – known as a double pit – may be set up at that point. A double pit is required for championships and recommended for other events.

5B3. In the equipment pits, the race course and the pit lane shall be separated and distinctly marked out, by tape at the very least. *The pit lane shall be a minimum of 3 meters wide at all points.*

STANDARD CONFIGURATION OF A DOUBLE PIT AREA

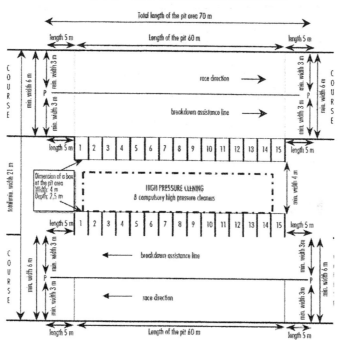

5B4. The equipment pits shall be sign-posted and precisely marked by means of a yellow flag at the beginning and the end of where the course is divided between the race and pit lanes.

5B5. Adjacent to the pit lane shall be an area with a minimum depth of 2 meters reserved for mechanics.

5B6. In championship events, a supply of water for cleaning equipment shall be available in the immediate vicinity of the equipment pits. The water supply and connections for high-pressure cleaning equipment shall be made freely available.

5C. Equipment changes

5C1. A rider may use the pit lane only to change a bicycle or wheel.

5C2. Changing of equipment shall be done at the same point with no advance in the rider's position.

5C3. A rider passing the pit entrance and continuing beyond the pit exit (yellow flagged area) may not enter that pit, but must continue around the course to the next pit. A rider not passing the pit exit, may enter that pit after dismounting and walking backwards on the course to the pit entrance.

5C4. The exchanging of wheels or bicycles between riders shall be forbidden.

5D. Starting

5D1. The riders shall assemble in the roll-call zone a maximum of 10 minutes before the start.

5D2. For championships the call up order shall be listed on the race announcement, information pamphlet, or at registration.

5D3. Any rider causing a false start shall be disqualified.

5E. Duration of races

5E1. The length of the race may be specified by number of laps or by time.

5E2. In events based on time, the number of laps to be ridden shall be determined on the basis of the time of the first rider to complete 2 full laps. From the 3rd lap on, the laps to go will be displayed at the finish line.

5F. Abandons

5F1. Riders dropping out shall immediately remove their body number and leave the course and may not cross the finish line.

5G. Finish

5G1. Any rider lapped before the last lap shall leave the race (unless stated differently prior to the race); if the lapping takes place after the midpoint of the race the rider shall be given a place. Lapped riders who are permitted to remain in the race will all finish on the same lap as the leader and will be placed according to the number of laps they are down and then their position at the finish.

5G2. In championship events a rider who is lapped during the final lap of the race shall be stopped at the beginning of the finish line area and shall be classified in accordance with their placing without crossing the finish line.

5H. In-race communication

5H1. The use of radios is forbidden

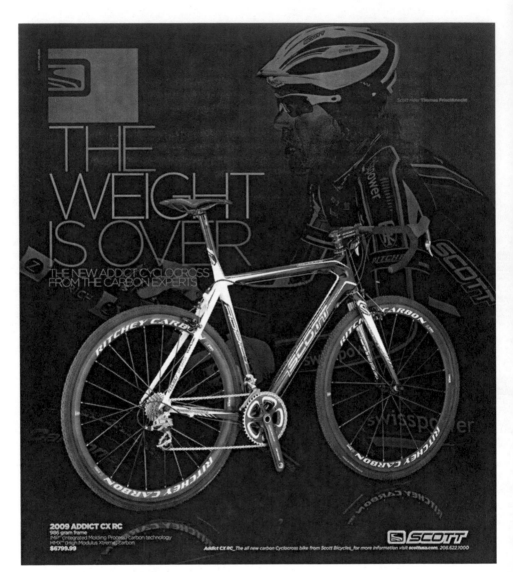

THE WEIGHT IS OVER

THE NEW ADDICT CYCLOCROSS
FROM THE CARBON EXPERTS

2009 ADDICT CX RC
986 gram frame
IMP™ (Integrated Molding Process) carbon technology
HMX™ (High Modulus Xtreme) carbon
$6799.99

Addict CX RC_The all new carbon Cyclocross bike from Scott Bicycles, for more information visit **scottusa.com.** *208.622.1000*

RIVAL - 2149 grams

Leap Lighter

"If I were equipping my own cyclocross bike, (SRAM) Rival would be my group of choice."

Matt Pacocha
VeloNews magazine technical editor

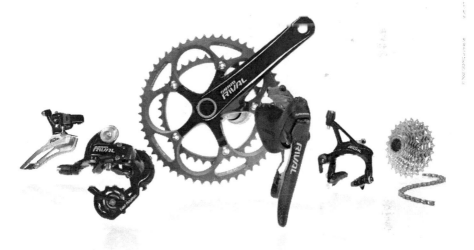

UPDATED for 2009!

The 2009 RIVAL gruppo sets the standard for performance level 10 speed! Now featuring critical trickle down upgrades from our revolutionary RED group, like structural carbon fiber, reach adjust control levers and faster shifting, New Rival is poised to set a new high water mark for performance road bikes.

Featuring enhanced blade shapes and exclusive adjustable ergonomics able to match any hand size, RIVALs new controls also inherit "Zero Loss" travel front shifting from RED, offering the serious road rider increased speed, quickness and accuracy. At just over 320grams per pair, in new slimming black and carbon wrap, these shifters set the standard for competition level and durable controls.

SRAM.

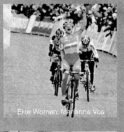
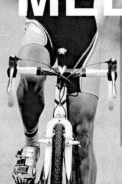
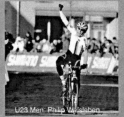
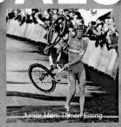
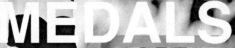
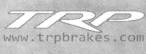

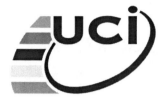

Union
Cycliste
Internationale

Cyclocross Rules

Reprinted with permission from Union Cycliste Internationale

(version on 1.07.09)

PART 5 CYCLO-CROSS RACES

TABLE OF CONTENTS

PART 5 CYCLO-CROSS RACES

Chapter CYCLO-CROSS EVENTS

§ 1 General Rules

Participation

5.1.001 Except where provided otherwise for the masters category, the category which will be applied for entries to races for the entire season is the category to which the rider will belong on 1 January of the following calendar year.

Men under 23 years
(N) Except in the UCI world championships, UCI world cup **events, when those include a separate men under 23** event and, at the discretion of national federations, national championships, men under 23 can ride the event for men elite, even if a separate event is being run for Under 23 riders.

Women
Women Juniors and women elite shall ride in the same events.

Masters
All riders who hold a Masters licence may ride in the **masters world championships** with the following exceptions:
1. Any rider who has ridden in the **UCI** world championships, continental championships or **UCI** world cup during the current season.
2. Any rider, who has been a member, during the current season, of a team registered with the UCI.
3. During the current season, any rider classified in **the** UCI individual cyclo-cross classification published following the national championships in Europe.

(text modified on 1.09.99; 1.09.04; 1.09.06; 1.09.08).

5.1.002 A rider ranked in the top 50 of the UCI cyclo-cross classification may not take part in national events in a country other than that of his national federation.

(text introduced on 1.09.04).

Race Programme - technical guide

5.1.003 The programme - technical guide must be written in French or English and in the official local language(s) **and include at least the following information:**
- **the special regulations for the race;**
- **schedule and times of races;**
- **the prize list;**
- **description and detailed map of the circuit, showing the circuit length and profile, the start and finish, the pit area and the obstacles;**
- **the location of the secretariat, accreditation issue point, the press room, and antidoping control location;**
- **timing and where applicable photo-finish installations;**
- **policing, security and emergency medical arrangements.**

(text modified on 1.09.04; 1.09.08).

Calendar

5.1.004 International cyclo-cross races are registered on the international calendar in accordance with the folowing classification:
- **UCI** *world championships: (CM)*
- **UCI cyclo-cross** world cup (WC)
- world masters championships (WMC)
- continental championships (CC)
- class 1 events (C1)
- class 2 events (C2)
- **events in the class women (CWE)**
- **events in the class men under 23 (CMU)**
- **events in the class men juniors (CMJ)**

The allocation of classes shall be carried out annually by the UCI management committee.

However, an event will only given class 1 status if the previous season's race had **at least** 10 foreign starters, representing at least 5 different nationalities.
A new event may only be added to the international calendar in class 2.

(article introduced on 1.09.06, text modified on 1.09.08).

Protection of the dates
UCI world championships

5.1.005 No other international cyclo-cross event may be organised on the days of the **UCI** world championships.

UCI world cup
No class 1 event may be held on the same day as a UCI world cup event.
No class 2 event may be held on the same day as a UCI world cup event in the same country.

(article introduced on 1.09.06; text modified on 1.09.08).

Technical delegate

5.1.006 At the **UCI** world championships, **UCI** world cup events and continental championships a technical delegate is appointed by the UCI.

Without prejudice to the responsibility of the organiser, the technical delegate shall supervise the preparation of the technical aspects of the event and shall serve as a link with UCI headquarters in this respect.

(article introduced on 1.09.06).

5.1.007 If an event is promoted at a new venue, the technical delegate must carry out an inspection well in advance to take the necessary measurements. The inspection will include the course, the distance, determine the double pit area, installations and the security. He will meet the organiser and prepare an inspection report without delay **for submission to the UCI cyclo-cross sports coordinator.**

He must be on site prior to the first **official** training session and **must** carry out an inspection of the venue and course in conjunction with the organiser and **the president of the commissaires' panel.** He shall coordinate the technical preparations for the event and shall ensure that the recommendations made in the inspection report are implemented. The definitive version of the course and any changes, if this is the case, shall be the responsibility of the technical delegate. **Where a technical delegate does not have to be appointed under article 5.1.006, this task shall fall to the president of the commissaires' panel.**

The technical delegate shall attend the team managers' meetings.

(article introduced on 1.09.06; text modified on 1.09.08).

Security

5.1.008 A zone of at least 100 metres before and 50 metres after the finish line will be protected with barriers. It will be accessible only to organisational staff, the riders, paramedics, team managers and accredited press. The organiser must strictly control access to this zone.

Adjacent parts of the course where riders pass in both directions must be separated by a safety net. The safety nets used must have no openings greater than 1 cm x 1 cm.

For events where large crowds are expected, on technical parts of the course, a safety area must be provided between the spectators and the course, as shown below:

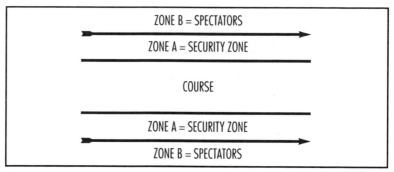

The Zone A sections must be minimum 75 cm wide.

The use of dangerous items along the course, such as fencing wire (barbed or otherwise) and metal stakes (including those used for advertising banners) is forbidden. The course must also be routed away from any item which presents danger to the riders.

From 5 minutes before the start of the race, the course may not be ridden by anyone other than the riders in the race.

The organiser must provide at least 4 crossing points for spectators on the course. The crossings must be marshalled on each side.

The race organiser must provide enough marshals to ensure the safety of the riders and spectators during competition and official training sessions.

(text modified on 1.09.04; 1.09.08).

5.1.008 **First aid**
bis At least one ambulance and one basic first aid post are required at all races.

For each event, at least one (1) doctor and at least four (4) people qualified to perform first aid under the laws of the country shall be present at the event.

(text modified on 1.09.04; 1.09.08).

Inflatable arches
5.1.009 The use of inflatable arches **which cross** the course is forbidden.

(article introduced on 1.02.07; text modified on 1.09.08).

Installations
5.1.010 The judge's stand at the finish must be covered and preferably located on the left of the course.

The organiser shall provide at least four radio sets to the commissaires' panel. These radio sets must have one channel reserved for the sole use of the commissaires' panel and another with which it is possible to contact the organiser.

(text modified on 1.09.99; 1.09.04).

5.1.011 The organiser must provide riders with a heated room, showers with hot and cold water and a water supply for cleaning of equipment. These installations must be no more than 2 km from the finish line.

Course

5.1.012 A cyclo-cross course shall include road, country and forest paths and meadowland alternating in such a way as to ensure changes in the pace of the race and allowing riders to recuperate after difficult sections.

[2nd paragraph abrogated on 1.08.00].

5.1.013 The course shall be usable in all circumstances, whatever the weather conditions.

Clay or easily flooded areas and agricultural land should be avoided..

5.1.014 A maximum of 5 events may be run on one course on the same day.

(text modified on 1.09.04).

5.1.015 The organiser must take steps to avoid damage to the course by spectators.

Before the start of each race, the organiser must check the condition of the course and carry out any repairs required.

For the UCI world championships, the UCI world cup events and the national championships, a parallel course is required for sections of the course which deteriorate easily.

(text modified on 1.09.99; 1.09.03 ; 1.09.04; 1.07.09).

5.1.016 **(moved last paragraph to article 5.1.008 on 1.09.08).**

5.1.017 The course must form a closed circuit of a minimum length of 2.5 km and maximum 3.5 km, of which at least 90% shall be ridable.

(text modified on 1.09.99; 1.09.04).

5.1.018 The course must be at least 3 metres wide throughout and clearly marked and protected on both sides.

(text modified on 1.09.99; 1.09.04; 1.09.08).

Call-up zone

5.1.019 An assembly area for starters (call-up zone) shall be provided and marked off behind the start line (see **Appendix** 1).

Eight lanes with a width of 75 cm and a length of 10 m shall be marked out on the ground at right angles to the start line in order to facilitate organising the riders into starting order (see **Appendix** 1).

(text modified on 1.09.99; 1.09.04; 1.09.06).

Start section

5.1.020 The start section must be on firm ground, and preferably on surfaced road. It must have a length of at least 200 metres and a width of at least 6 metres. It must be as straight as possible and not include any descent. The first narrowing or obstacle after the start section may not be abrupt, it must be such as to allow all the riders to pass easily. The **angle of the** first corner must be greater than **90 degrees. The start banner shall be erected at least 2.5 m above the ground over the start line and shall cover the whole width of the start section.**

(text modified on 1.09.03; 1.09.04; 1.09.06; 1.09.08).

Finish section

5.1.021 The finish section must run straight for at least 100 metres. The width must be at least 6 metres for UCI world championships, UCI world cup events and events in class 1, and at least 4 metres for other events. The section must be flat or uphill. **The finish banner shall be erected at least 2.5 m above the ground over the finish line and shall cover the whole width of the finish section.**

(text modified on 1.09.04; 1.09.06; 1.09.08).

Obstacles

5.1.022 The start and finish sections must be free of obstacles.

(text modified on 1.09.04).

5.1.023 The course may include no more than six obstacles. Obstacle shall mean any part of the course which is likely to require riders to dismount.

The length of an obstacle may not exceed 80 metres. The total length of obstacles may not exceed 10% of the course.

Sand sections especially constructed for the event are forbidden. The natural aspect of the course must be respected.

Descents of flights of steps may not be used.

(text modified on 1.08.00; 1.09.04; 1.07.09).

5.1.024 The course may include a single section of planks. This obstacle must consist of two planks placed 4 metres apart. The planks must be solid for their entire height and not made of metal. They must have a height of 40 cm and extend the entire width of the course. In races for men juniors and women, it is recommended that a parallel course avoiding this obstacle should be used.

In the event that the course is abnormally slippery, the plank section must be removed on the decision of the president of the commissaires' panel in consultation with the organiser and, should he be present, the UCI technical delegate or the cyclo-cross **sport** coordinator.

(text modified on 1.08.00; 1.09.03; 1.09.04; 1.09.08).

5.1.025 The course may pass over bridges or footbridges as long as they are at least 3 metres wide and have protective barriers on both sides. Bridges or footbridges shall be covered with an anti-slip surface (matting, mesh or anti-slip paint).

In addition a separate footbridge for spectators must be provided.

(text modified on 1.09.99; 1.09.04).

Pit areas
5.1.026 The pit area is the part of the course where riders can change wheels or bicycles.

(text modified on 1.09.04).

5.1.027 The pit areas must be straight and may not include any obstacle. They must be located on a part of the course where the speed is not high, excluding gravelled sections and descents.

(text modified on 1.09.04).

5.1.028 The double pit area (see **Appendix** 2) is compulsory for UCI world championships, UCI world cup events, national championships and events in class 1.

If it is not possible to design a course such that a double pit area as per article 5.1.029 can be set up, the event may only be organised with the prior consent of the cyclo-cross commission to set up two single pits (see **Appendix** 3).

(text modified on 1.09.04).

5.1.029 The double pit area must be set up in an area where two sections of the course are close enough together and the distance along the course between the successive pits is more or less equal each way.

(text modified on 1.09.04).

5.1.030 For UCI world championships, the location for the double pit area shall be set by the UCI technical delegate.

(text introduced on 1.09.04).

5.1.031 In events other than those covered by article 5.1.028, the organiser must make provision for a double pit area or two single pit areas located at suitable distances around the course.

(text modified on 1.09.04).

5.1.032 For the whole length of the pits the racing lane and the pit lane must be separated, using barriers and marker tape.

The pit area must be signalled and marked precisely with a yellow flag at the beginning and the end of the separation between the two lanes.

(text modified on 1.08.00; 1.09.04).

5.1.033 At the side of the pit lane a zone at least 2 metres deep shall be set aside for riders' mechanics and their equipment.

(text modified on 1.08.00; 1.02.07; 26.06.07).

5.1.034 In double pit areas provision must be made for a water supply for cleaning of equipment. For single pit areas the water supply must be in the immediate proximity such that mechanics do not have to cross the course to access it.

If a water tank or connections for high pressure cleaning apparatus are provided, they must be made freely available.

At UCI world championships and UCI world cup events the organiser must provide eight high-pressure cleaners in the pit area.

(text modified on 1.09.98; 1.09.04).

Boxes

5.1.035 *At UCI world championships and UCI world cup events the pit areas must be at least 70 metres long.*

Along the pit lane provision must be made for 12 to 15 boxes marked off by barriers with a width of 4 metres (see **Appendix** 2).

For **class** 1 events the pits must be at least 60 metres long and at least 12 boxes must be provided.

Only two accredited assistants per rider shall be allowed in the box of this rider.

(text modified on 1.08.00; 1.09.03; 1.09.04; 1.02.07).

5.1.036 **Allocation of boxes**
The pit boxes are allocated at the meeting between the commissaires' panel and the team leaders, **as follows:**

A. UCI world championships:
Separately for each category on the basis of the most recently published UCI cyclo-cross rankings by nation for the category concerned.

B. UCI world cup
● **1st event:**
Separately for each category on the basis of the final UCI cyclo-cross classification by nation of the previous season for the category concerned;
● **Other events:**
Separately for each category on the basis of the most recently published UCI cyclo-cross classification by nation for the category concerned.

The allocation of boxes to teams that do not feature in **the relevant classification** shall be by drawing lots.

The team leaders shall select their preferred box in the order **thus determined.**

(text modified on 1.09.9; 1.09.05; 1.09.08; 1.07.09).

5.1.037 **[article abrogated on 1.09.08].**

Equipment changes
5.1.038 A rider may only take the pit lane to change his bicycle or a wheel.

(text modified on 1.09.04).

5.1.039 Equipment changes must be carried out within the confines of the pit lane and at the same point.

[2nd paragraph abrogated on 1.09.05].

A rider who has passed the end of the pit area must continue to the following pit area for any bicycle or wheel change. A rider who is still in the racing lane may enter the pit lane as long as he retraces his route in the racing lane and enters the other lane at its start without obstructing other competitors.

(text modified on 1.08.00; 1.09.03; 1.09.04).

5.1.040   Changes of wheel or bicycle between riders are forbidden.

5.1.041   **Attendants**
Each rider may be accompanied by a paramedical assistant and two mechanics.

The paramedical assistant and the mechanics must be provided by the organiser with a free accreditation, which gives them access to the area reserved for them by virtue of their office.

The accreditations must be distributed outside the circuit, in a clearly indicated place.

(article introduced on 26.06.07).

 § 2   Event procedure

Starting order
5.1.042   The riders shall assemble in the call-up zone **defined in article 5.1.019** at least 10 minutes before the start.

Riders must wait for the start with at least one foot on the ground, or be penalised by being sent back to the last place in their start lane.

(text modified on 1.10.02; 1.09.08).

5.1.043   **The start order of events is determined as follows:**
A) UCI world championships:
   - *Men elite and women:*
     As per the most recently published UCI cyclo-cross individual classification of the current season;
   - *Men under 23 and men juniors:*
     1. The first 16 of the individual classification of the last UCI world cup standings men under 23 and the first 16 of the individual classification of the last UCI world cup standings men juniors.
     Then:
     2. The order of the riders for each country must be fixed and communicated by the national federations;
     3. The countries are ranked on the basis of the classification by nation of the concerned category from the UCI world championships of the previous season;
     4. Taking each country in turn, a place is allocated to the next rider in sequence;
     5. Federations which do not appear in the classification by nations specified above shall, on the basis of the same rotation system, take the last places, in an order determined by the drawing of lots by the commissaires' panel.

B) UCI world cup:
- Men elite and women:
  1. **1st event:**
  As per the final UCI individual cyclo-cross classification of the **previous** season.
  2. Other events:
  As per the last published UCI individual cyclo-cross classification of the current season.

- Men under 23 and men juniors:
  1. **1st event:**
  by nations in rotation as per article 5.1.**043 for the UCI world championships** (points 2 to 5).
  2. **other events:**
  by nations in rotation as per article 5.1.043 for the UCI world championships (points 1 to 5).
  The riders of the B team of the national federation of the organiser permitted under article 5.3.006 paragraph 3 **shall take the last positions.**

C) Continental championships:
- **Men elite (outside Europe) and women:**
  As per the most recently published UCI cyclo-cross individual classification of the current season.
- **Men under 23 and men juniors:**
  By nations in rotation as per article 5.1.043 for the UCI world championships (points 2 to 5).

D) Other events:
- Men elite, women, men under 23 **and men juniors:**
  As per the most recently published UCI cyclo-cross individual classification for the current season **for the category concerned.**
  If no classification has yet been published for the current season, the start order will be determined by the final UCI individual cyclo-cross classification for the previous season.

(text modified on 1.09.99; 1.10.02; 1.09.03; 1.09.04; 1.02.07; 26.06.07; 1.09.08; 1.07.09).

5.1.044 [article abrogated on 1.09.08].

5.1.045 [article abrogated on 1.09.08].

Allocation of race numbers

5.1.046 *The allocation of race numbers at UCI world championships and UCI world cup events shall be as follows:*
- *Race numbers in sequence from 1 **upwards** to the country of the world champion of the preceding season;*
- ***Race number 1 shall only be allocated to the reigning world champion of the category concerned;***
- *The other race numbers are issued to nations on the basis of their classification in the UCI world championships of the preceding season;*
- *For nations not ranked or not having taken part in the UCI world championship the preceding season, the allocation shall be by drawing lots by the commissaires' panel.*

(text modified on 1.09.99; 1.09.03; 1.09.04; 1.09.06; 1.09.08).

False start

5.1.047 Riders who cause a false start shall be pulled out of the race.

In case of a false start, a new call up procedure and gridding will be done.

(text modified on 1.09.06).

Duration of events

5.1.048 The duration of events must be as close as possible to:
- 40 minutes for women's events
- 40 minutes for juniors men's events
- 50 minutes for under 23 men's events
- 60 minutes for the elite men's events and for events in which elite and men under 23 ride together.

During UCI world championships and UCI world cup events the elite men events will be between 60 and 70 minutes.

(text modified on 1.09.01; 1.09.06).

Last lap

5.1.049 The last lap of the race shall be announced by the bell.

(text modified on 1.09.06).

Retirement

5.1.050 A rider who retires must leave the course immediately and does not have the right to cross the finish line. **He shall be listed in the results as «DNF» («did not finish») and shall not be awarded any points for this event.**

(text modified on 1.09.04; 1.09.08).

Classification

5.1.051 Each rider lapped before the final lap must leave the race the next time they cross the finish line. **He shall be listed in the results with his total number of laps behind the winner.**

A rider who is lapped on the final lap shall be stopped at the beginning of the finishing straight line and shall be given a placing on the basis of his position.

(text modified on 1.09.98; 1.09.04; 1.09.08).

5.1.052 All riders who cross the finish line after the winner shall have finished the race and will be given a placing on the basis of their position.

5.1.053 *At the UCI world championships, a classification by nation shall be drawn up on the basis of the places of the first three riders from each nation. Nation with two riders finishing shall be ranked after those with three. The nation with one rider finishing shall be ranked after those with two.*
The classification by nation shall not be used for a world champion's title.

(text modified on 1.09.03).

Official ceremony

5.1.054 The official ceremony shall take place immediately after the last rider has finished and shall take no longer than 10 minutes.

5.1.055 Those involved in the official ceremony are permitted to wear additional clothing.

Results

5.1.056 **The president of the commissaires' panel is required to send the full results immediately to UCI headquarters by e-mail or, if it is not available, by fax. All National Federations must immediately notify the UCI of any fact or decision which would result in a change to the points awarded to a rider.**

In the event of a failure to fulfil these obligates, the UCI Management Committee may relegate the event in question to a lower class or exclude it from the world or continental calendar, without prejudice to the penalties applicable under the Regulations.

(text modified on 1.09.04; 1.09.05; 1.09.06; 1.09.08).

5.1.057 (N) The organiser's national federation shall notify the UCI as fast as possible of any change to the result reported by the organiser.

Cancellation

5.1.058   In the event of difficult weather conditions (e.g. strong winds, heavy snowfall, temperatures below −15°) the president of the commissaires' panel may decide to cancel the event, after consulting the UCI technical delegate in case of need and the organizer.

(text modified on 1.09.99; 1.09.04).

In-race communications

5.1.059   The use of radio links or other remote means of communication with riders is forbidden.

(text introduced on 1.09.04).

Chapter UCI CYCLO-CROSS CLASSIFICATION

5.2.001 The UCI shall draw up an annual individual classification of riders who take part in international cyclo-cross events:
- **a joint classification for men elite and men under 23;**
- **a classification for women;**
- **a classification for men juniors.**

The classification shall be called the UCI cyclo-cross classification.

(text modified on 1.09.04; 1.09.08).

5.2.002 The UCI cyclo-cross classification is the exclusive property of the UCI.

(text modified on 1.09.04).

5.2.003 The UCI cyclo-cross classification is drawn up annually by summing the points won by each rider in international cyclo-cross events in the period from 1 September to 28 or 29 February.

In case of riders placed equal in the ranking, their place in the most recent ranking of the season, considering only places being rewarded with UCI points will decide between them in the following order:
1. UCI world championships
2. UCI world cup events
3. **continental championships**
4. **national championships**
5. class 1 events
6. class 2 events
7. **events in the class women, men under 23 and men juniors.**

(text modified on 1.09.04; 1.09.05; 1.09.06; 1.09.08).

5.2.004 The events are classified into **17** categories on the basis of the number of points to be awarded:
a. UCI world championships men elite and UCI world championships women
b. UCI world championships men under 23
c. UCI world championships men juniors
d. UCI world cup events men elite and women
e UCI world cup events men under 23
f. UCI world cup events men juniors
g. continental championships men elite (except Europe), women
h. continental championships men under 23
i. continental championships men juniors
j. national championships men elite and women

k. national championships men under 23
l. national championships men juniors
m. events in class 1
n. events in class 2
o. events **in the class** women
p. events in the class men under 23 (where there is a separate event for men elite)
q. events in the class men juniors

(text modified on 1.09.99; 1.09.03; 1.09.04; 1.09.06; 1.09.08).

5.2.005 The classification of events in the categories specified in points d to i and from m to q of article 5.2.004 is carried out annually by the UCI management committee.

(text modified on 1.09.03; 1.09.04; 1.09.06; 1.09.08).

5.2.006 The number of points to be awarded in each event is mentioned in the attachment at this chapter:
For events in the categories below, only the best results of each rider shall be taken into account:
- class 1 events: the best 6 results of each rider;
- class 2 events: the best 5 results of each rider;
- **events in the women's class: the best 12 results of each rider;**
- **events in the juniors men's class: the best 6 results of each rider.**

(text modified on 1.08.00; 1.09.03; 1.09.04; 1.09.05; 1.09.06; 1.09.08; 1.07.09).

5.2.007 [article abrogated on 1.09.08].

5.2.008 (moved to article 5.1.056 on 1.09.08).

5.2.009 **A UCI individual cyclo-cross classification is** drawn up after UCI world cup round, the UCI world championships, the national championships and at the end of the season (the end of February). It is used for the start order of riders in the international events given in **article 5.1.043.**

(text modified on 1.09.98; 1.09.04; 1.09.05; 1.09.08).

5.2.010 At the same time a **UCI cyclo-cross** classification by nation for **men elite**, a UCI cyclo-cross classification by nation for women, **a UCI cyclo-cross classification by nation men under 23 and a UCI cyclo-cross classification by nation men juniors** are drawn up by totaling the points of the three first classified riders of each nation.

In case of nations placed equal in the ranking, the place of its best rider in the individual ranking will break the tie.

(text modified on 1.09.98; 1.09.03; 1.09.04; 1.09.05; 1.09.08; 1.07.09).

5.2.011 [article abrogated on 1.09.08].

5.2.012 [article abrogated on 1.09.08].

5.2.013 (article moved to article 1.3.058b).

Chapter **UCI CYCLO-CROSS WORLD CUP**

5.3.001   The UCI cyclo-cross world cup is the exclusive property of the UCI.

(text modified on 1.09.04).

5.3.002   The UCI **cyclo-cross** world cup is contested over a number of events in at least 6 different coun-tries. These events shall be selected annually by the UCI Management Committee as per the proce-dure set out in the bidding procedure manual and the **cyclo-cross** world cup organisation guide.

(text modified on 1.09.99; 1.09.04).

5.3.003   The designation of an event as a UCI **cyclo-cross** world cup event shall be subject to the signing of a contract by the organiser with the UCI governing inter alia the audio-visual broadcasting rights, marketing rights and the practical organisation of the race.

5.3.004   Article transferred to art. 5.1.005.

(text modified on 1.09.06).

Participation
5.3.005   UCI **cyclo-cross** world cup events shall be organised for elite men, women, men under 23, and men juniors.

The rounds of the UCI cyclo-cross world cup for men elite, women, men under 23 and men juniors will be specified on the UCI web site.

Entries for riders shall be submitted to the UCI by the federation of their nationality.

(text modified on 1.10.02; 1.09.03; 1.09.04; 1.09.08).

5.3.006   In **UCI cyclo-cross** world cup events for elite men and women, each federation may enter 8 riders. The federations concerned may additionally enter the reigning world champions and the leaders of the last UCI **cyclo-cross world cup** classification published **before the opening date for entries.**

No points for the **UCI cyclo-cross** world cup for men under 23 are awarded for results in elite men's events.

In **UCI cyclo-cross** world cup events for men under 23 and men juniors, each federation may enter 6 riders. The federations concerned may additionally enter the reigning world champion. The national federation of the organising country may register two national team of 6 riders (team A and team B) for the men under 23 category as well as for the men juniors category.

In accordance with article. 1.3.059, **all** riders **in the men under 23 and men juniors categories** must wear national team clothing.

A table listing the opening and closing dates for entries will be published on the UCI website.

(text modified on 1.09.99; 1.10.02; 1.09.03; 1.09.04; 26.06.07; 1.09.08).

5.3.007 **[article abrogated on 1.09.08].**

5.3.008 **The national federations must submit entries to the UCI for their riders no later than ten days before each event of the UCI cyclo-cross world cup, including the riders for the B team of the national federation of the country of the organiser.**

Without prejudice to article 13.1.070, the **entry** will not be accepted if the hotel where the riders will be staying is not specified at the time of registration.

In the event of a late entry, the national federation shall be liable to pay a fine of 150 Swiss francs per rider.

(text modified on 1.09.04; 1.09.05; 1.09.08).

5.3.009 A rider **for whom an entry has been submitted to the UCI under article 5.3.008** for a UCI **cyclo-cross** world cup event may not ride any other cyclo-cross event in any category whatsoever on the same day. Should he do so, he shall be subject to disqualification and a fine of between 500 and 3000 Swiss francs.

(text modified on 1.09.99; 1.10.02; 1.09.04; 1.09.08).

Clothing
5.3.010 Article transferred to art. 1.3.058 b.

Official ceremony
5.3.011 The official ceremony shall be held within 5 minutes after the winner of **each category** finishes. **The first 3 riders in the race and the leader of the general classification of the UCI cyclo-cross world cup must attend the podium.**

(text modified on 1.09.98; 1.09.08).

5.3.012 After the official ceremony the first 3 riders in the event shall be required to attend the press room in the company of the organiser.

(text modified on 1.09.04).

Classifications

1. Men elite:

5.3.013 A UCI **individual cyclo-cross** world cup classification will be drawn up for the category **men** elite, **for which points will be awarded to the first 50 riders in each race in accordance with the following scale:**

Place	Points	Place	Points
1	80	26	25
2	70	27	24
3	65	28	23
4	60	29	22
5	55	30	21
6	50	31	20
7	48	32	19
8	46	33	18
9	44	34	17
10	42	35	16
11	40	36	15
12	39	37	14
13	38	38	13
14	37	39	12
15	36	40	11
16	35	41	10
17	34	42	9
18	33	43	8
19	32	44	7
20	31	45	6
21	30	46	5
22	29	47	4
23	28	48	3
24	27	49	2
25	26	50	1

2. Women, men under 23, men juniors:

Separate **UCI individual cyclo-cross world cup classifications** will be drawn up for the categories **women,** men under 23 and men juniors, for which points will be awarded to the first 30 riders in each race in accordance with the following scale:

Place	Points	Place	Points
1	60	16	15
2	50	17	14
3	45	18	13
4	40	19	12
5	35	20	11
6	30	21	10
7	28	22	9
8	26	23	8
9	24	24	7
10	22	25	6
11	20	26	5
12	19	27	4
13	18	28	3
14	17	29	2
15	16	30	1

Riders tying on points **will be** ranked by **the greatest number of 1st places, 2nd places, etc. taking account only of places for which points are awarded for the UCI cyclo-cross world cup. If they are still tied, the points scored in most recent event shall be used to separate them.**

(text modified on 1.09.99; 1.09.02; 1.09.04; 1.09.05; 1.09.08).

5.3.014 *[abrogated on 1.09.04].*

5.3.015 [abrogated on 1.09.03].

5.3.016 *[abrogated on 1.09.04].*

5.3.017 [abrogated on 1.09.04].

Prizes

5.3.018 The scale of prizes for the individual classification for each event will be determined by the UCI management committee.

At least three months before the event, the organiser shall provide a bank guarantee to the organiser's national federation equal to the total prize fund.

In the event that a prize or prizes are unpaid, the event shall not be considered as a **UCI cyclo-cross** world cup event the following season.

(text modified on 1.09.99; 1.09.04).

5.3.019 The UCI shall award prizes to the first 25 men elite and the first 10 women of the final individual classification of the UCI cyclo-cross world cup, with values which will be set out in the financial obligations of the UCI.

(article introduced on 1.09.08).

5.3.020 [abrogated on 1.09.99].

5.3.021 [abrogated on 1.09.04].

Trophies

5.3.022 The UCI shall award a trophy to the first three of the final classification of the UCI **cyclo-cross** world cup **in each category.**

(text modified on 1.09.02; 1.09.03; 1.09.04;1.09.06; 1.09.08).

Leader's skinsuit

5.3.023 **For each category, the** UCI shall award a leader's skinsuit to the **leader** in the individual classification **of** the UCI cyclo-cross world cup.
In all rounds other than the first the leader shall be required to wear the leader's skinsuit in all the UCI cyclo-cross world cup events.
The leader's skinsuit may only be worn at rounds of the UCI cyclo-cross world cup, and in no other event.

(text modified on 1.09.98; 1.09.04; 1.09.05; 1.09.08).

5.3.024 Article transferred to art. 1.3.058 b.

Appendix 1
Call-up zone

STANDARD CONFIGURATION OF A START AREA

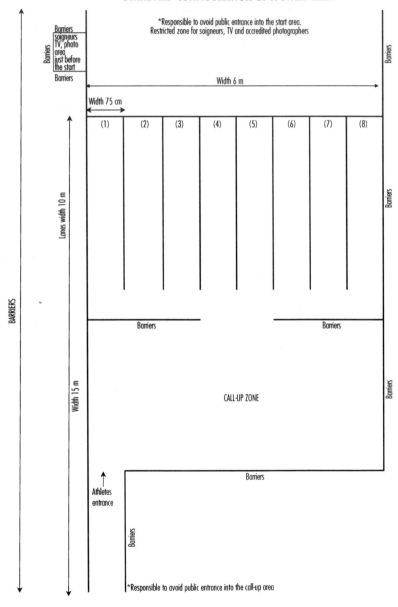

Appendix 2
Double pit area

STANDARD CONFIGURATION OF A DOUBLE PIT AREA

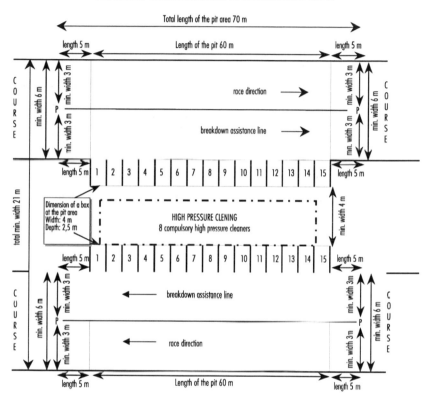

Appendix 3
Single pit area

STANDARD CONFIGURATION OF A PIT AREA

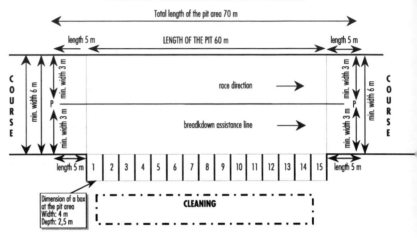

Appendix 4
UCI points table

Place	UCI WORLD CHAMPIONSHIPS			UCI WORLD CUP			CONTINENTAL CHAMPIONSHIPS			NATIONAL CHAMPIONSHIPS			Class 1	Class 2	Class Women	Class MU	Class MJ
	Men Elite Women	Men U23	Men Junior	Men Elite Women	Men U23*	Men Juniors*	Men Elite Women	Men U23*	Men Juniors*	Men Elite Women	Men U23*	Men Juniors*	Elite	Elite	Women	Men U23	Men Juniors
1	400	200	60	300	100	30	150	100	30	120	60	20	60	30	20	20	10
2	360	150	40	260	60	20	100	60	20	60	30	15	40	20	15	15	6
3	320	120	30	220	40	15	70	40	15	50	25	12	30	15	12	12	4
4	280	100	25	190	30	12	50	30	12	40	20	10	25	12	10	10	2
5	240	90	20	170	25	10	30	25	10	30	15	8	20	10	8	8	1
6	200	80	18	150	20	8	20	20	8	25	13	5	18	8	5	5	x
7	190	70	16	140	17	6	17	17	6	20	10	4	16	6	4	4	
8	180	60	14	130	15	4	15	15	4	15	8	3	14	4	3	3	
9	170	55	12	120	12	2	12	12	2	10	5	2	12	2	2	2	
10	160	50	10	110	10	1	10	10	1	5	3	1	10	1	1	1	
11	150	45	8	100	8	x	8	8	x	x	x	x	8	x	x	x	
12	140	40	6	90	6		6	6					6				
13	130	35	4	80	4		4	4					4				
14	120	30	2	75	2		2	2					2				
15	110	25	1	70	1		1	1					1				
16	100	20	x	65	x		x	x					x				
17	90	18		60													
18	80	16		57													
19	70	14		54													
20	60	12		51													
21	57	10		48													
22	54	9		46													
23	51	8		44													
24	48	7		42													
25	45	6		40													

Place	UCI WORLD CHAMPIONSHIPS Men Elite Women	Men U23	Men Junior	UCI WORLD CUP Men Elite Women	Men U23*	Men Juniors*	CONTINENTAL CHAMPIONSHIPS Men Elite Women	Men U23*	Men Juniors*	NATIONAL CHAMPIONSHIPS Men Elite Women	Men U23*	Men Juniors*	Class 1 Elite	Class 2 Elite	Class Women Women	Class MU Men U23	Class MJ Men Juniors
26	42	5		38													
27	39	4		36													
28	36	3		34													
29	33	2		32													
30	30	1		30													
31	28	x		29													
32	26			28													
33	24			27													
34	22			26													
35	20			25													
36	18			24													
37	16			23													
38	14			22													
39	12			21													
40	10			20													
41	5**			19													
42				18													
43				17													
44				16													
45				15													
46				14													
47				13													
48				12													
49				11													
50				10													
51				5**													

*in case of split event / ** amount of points for each ranked rider.

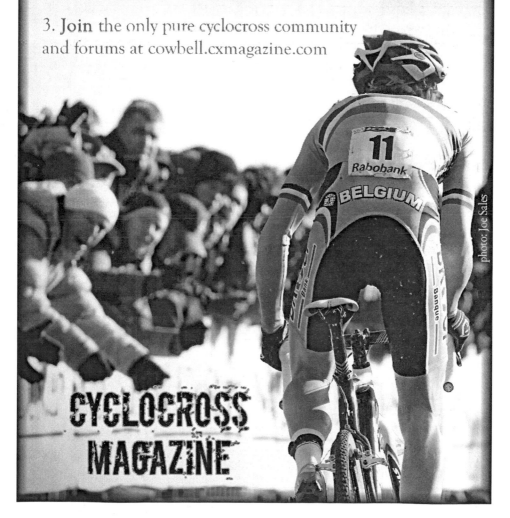

DON'T STOP NOW!

Take the three essential steps to continue your 'cross learning:

1. **Subscribe** to *Cyclocross Magazine* for in-depth training advice, reviews, rider interviews, 'cross culture pieces and more

2. **Visit** www.cxmagazine.com for the latest cyclocross news, race reports, photos and videos

3. **Join** the only pure cyclocross community and forums at cowbell.cxmagazine.com

photo: Joe Sales

CYCLOCROSS MAGAZINE

Contributors

Scott Hackett

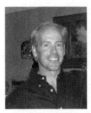 Scott has spent nearly all of his life involved in some sort of athletics, some at a high level and some just for the enjoyment and experience. This wide range of athletic experiences has taught him that you don't have to be "the best of the best" to benefit from top notch personalized coaching and conditioning programs like he has designed for national and world-class athletes. He's found that total beginners and recreational athletes almost always reap greater rewards from the experience of personal coach and trainer.

- Education, Present and Past Certifications

- BA Exercise Science, CSCS

- NSCA Certified Strength and Conditioning Specialist

- ASEP Master Level: Teaching Sport Skills, Sport Psychology, Sport Administration

- ASEP Leader level Coaching Principals

- ACE, AFFA Personal Trainer, Aerobics Instructor 1989-1995

- Former USA Cycling Elite Coaching License (Level 1) & Former Resident MTB Coach at the Olympic Training Center in Colorado Springs, CO

- Red Cross, First Responder, First Aid, CPR, AED

Beth Wrenn-Estes

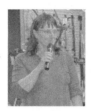 Beth has been involved in the sport of bicycle racing since 1973. Among her promotion credits are the 1987 Pan Am Trials, 1991 Junior Worlds, The Bob Cook Memorial/Mt. Evans Hill Climb (1981-1998) and the 1996 Olympic Games as Competition Manager for Cycling. Beth has also promoted many other events in Colorado since the mid-1970's.

Beth is a Category A International UCI Commissaire (Referee) obtaining her A in Belgium in 1988. She is also a Category 1/USA Cycling National Commissaire. Beth has worked as a referee both nationally and internationally since 1973 working all the major professional races in the 1980's and 1990's and being part of the officiating crew for all 13 years of the Coors Classic.

Beth's work with adolescents (Juniors) is her passion. It was she and Scott Mares that created the Mudskippers Junior Cyclocross Team. She was also the driving force for the creation of the Junior Camps, Juniors Ride Free, the First Bike Programs, and the Tom Danielson Junior Road Series while she was Executive Director for The American Cycling Association.

CPSIA information can be obtained at www.ICGtesting.com
Printed in the USA
BVOW041756250912

301314BV00006B/3/P